DSM-5® DIAGNOSIS IN THE SCHOOLS

Also Available

The First Session with Children and Adolescents: Conducting a Comprehensive Mental Health Evaluation
Alvin E. House

DSM-5® Diagnosis in the Schools

Renée M. Tobin
Alvin E. House

THE GUILFORD PRESS
New York London

A Division of Guilford Publications, Inc.
370 Seventh Avenue, Suite 1200, New York, NY 10001
www.guilford.com

Paperback edition 2020

Printed in the United States of America

This book is printed on acid-free paper.

Last digit is print number: 9 8 7 6 5 4 3

The authors have checked with sources believed to be reliable in their efforts to provide information that is complete and generally in accord with the standards of practice that are accepted at the time of publication. However, in view of the possibility of human error or changes in behavioral, mental health, or medical sciences, neither the authors, nor the editors and publisher, nor any other party who has been involved in the preparation or publication of this work warrants that the information contained herein is in every respect accurate or complete, and they are not responsible for any errors or omissions or the results obtained from the use of such information. Readers are encouraged to confirm the information contained in this book with other sources.

Library of Congress Cataloging-in-Publication Data

Tobin, Renée Margaret.
DSM-5 diagnosis in the schools / Renée M. Tobin, Alvin E. House.
pages cm
Includes bibliographical references and index.
ISBN 978-1-4625-2372-6 (hardback) ISBN 978-1-4625-4374-8 (paperback)
1. Child psychopathology—Diagnosis. 2. Adolescent psychopathology—Diagnosis. 3. Diagnostic and statistical manual of mental disorders.
I. House, Alvin E. II. Title.
RJ503.5.T63 2016
618.92′89075—dc23

2015016848

About the Authors

Renée M. Tobin, PhD, is Professor and Chair of the Department of Psychological Studies in Education at Temple University. She teaches graduate-level courses in social, emotional, and behavioral assessment; theories of counseling; consultation; and counseling techniques. She also supervises interns and advanced doctoral students providing assessment, consultation, and therapy for children and adolescents in school, clinic, and residential placement settings. Her primary research publications examine personality and social development, with a focus on promoting emotion regulation processes in youth.

Alvin E. House, PhD, is Professor Emeritus in the Department of Psychology at Illinois State University. His professional practice and research focus on applying assessment results in school, vocational, medical, and forensic consultations. Dr. House is the author of *The First Session with Children and Adolescents* and coauthor of a manual on observational assessment of children. His publications also include journal articles and book chapters on intellectual, personality, and neuropsychological testing.

Acknowledgments

We thank our spouses, Joel Schneider and Angie House, for their support and encouragement. We also thank our children, Ryan Tobin-Schneider, Tiechera Samuell, and Brannan House. Witnessing their development has added depth to our understanding of the processes of change and growth that we discuss in this book. Our family members also put up with long periods of unavailability while we worked to bring this book to fruition, and we are grateful. We thank the chair of our department, J. Scott Jordan, who recognizes the unique contributions of each member of our department and allowed us the space to follow our interests. We thank two graduate assistants, Kiera Dymit and Allyson Satterlee, for their efforts in gathering relevant materials for this book. Finally, we applaud the patience of our editor at The Guilford Press, Natalie Graham, who gently pushed this project to its completion.

Contents

1

Introduction

Purposes and Features of This Book

WHAT THIS BOOK IS—AND IS NOT—INTENDED TO DO

Efficient and accurate use of the fifth edition of the American Psychiatric Association's (2013b) *Diagnostic and Statistical Manual of Mental Disorders* (DSM-5) has become a necessary part of the professional duties of psychologists in a variety of clinical, rehabilitative, and youth service agencies. For several reasons, this development has extended into public school systems, where school psychologists are increasingly being asked to make DSM-5 diagnostic determinations. Research examining prevalence rates indicates that one in five youth has a mental health issue (Kessler et al., 2005, 2012). Consistent with these findings, Doll's (1996) review of epidemiological studies concluded with the statement that "a typical school of 1,000 students could be expected to have between 180 and 220 students with diagnosable psychiatric disorders" (p. 29). This book is intended to increase school-based practitioners' familiarity with DSM-5 and to bolster their confidence in using it within school settings. The use of DSM-5 is often made difficult by both the size of the text (806 pages presented in 20 chapters on disorders) and the complexity of the taxonomy (more than 300 diagnoses). Some of the rules and conventions adopted to bring increased structure and reliability to the system add further to the complexity of the document for novice users. These considerations, combined with timidity about using a "medical" system, may leave neophytes feeling totally confused and frustrated. This volume attempts to provide a broad understanding of the DSM-5 system—what it attempts to do, how it is organized, and how to use it most effectively to capture and communicate the unique features of youths' problems.

It is interesting to note a stylistic change in the most recent edition of the DSM. The editions between the first DSM publication in 1952 and the current version published in 2013 were indicated by Roman numerals (II, III, III-R, IV, IV-TR). The current version has changed to an Arabic numeral. The intent, clear in some of the associated Internet discussions, is to make subsequent "mini-revisions" easier, much like computer software is updated. We can probably anticipate seeing DSM-5.1 some time in the near future. Minor changes, largely typographical, have already occurred in electronic versions and print runs of DSM-5.

DSM can be viewed from several perspectives. One way is to think about it as if it were a language used to communicate about a particular topic: the vicissitudes and foibles of human existence. Good diagnostic practice, much like good writing, is to use this language to capture as completely and accurately as possible the difficulties faced by the particular youth you are evaluating. Like all languages, DSM changes over time, as a function of both our understanding of fundamentals of the human condition and of the culture and time in which we exist. Human life has changed in some ways over the past few centuries, and with these changes have come some shifts as well in the problems we experience; in many other respects the human experience is still as it was in our great-grandparents' time or in their great-grandparents' time, and many of the challenges seem constant over the ages.

This book does *not* take the place of DSM-5. Any psychologist who plans to use DSM-5 will need a copy of it (see the Professional Note). Several other books are available on using DSM-5; significant amounts of text in these volumes are often devoted to paraphrasing the DSM category definitions and diagnostic criteria. This repetition adds to the size and cost of these books, but it does not eliminate the need to have a copy of DSM-5. This volume, unlike these others, does not repeat or paraphrase DSM-5 categories. Instead, this book shows how the system is organized and how this organization relates to common presenting problems, as well as to other classification systems with which readers may be familiar.

Related to the issue of having a copy of DSM-5 available is the question of attempting to memorize the criteria. Various memory aids have been developed for previous diagnostic categories. For example, Reeves and Bullen (1995) published mnemonics for 10 of the DSM-IV Mental Disorders or syndromes: Major Depression, Mania, Dysthymia, Generalized Anxiety

Disorder, Posttraumatic Stress Disorder, Panic Attack, Anorexia Nervosa, Bulimia Nervosa, Delirium, and Borderline Personality Disorder. Although there are probably useful applications for such devices, in general we do not advise attempting to memorize diagnostic categories. There are several reasons for this recommendation, but a strong pragmatic one is the sheer number of categories and criteria in DSM-5. It is probably far more efficient to use the *Desk Reference to the Diagnostic Criteria from DSM-5* (American Psychiatric Association, 2013a) as a prompt or to develop one's own checklist than to try to learn dozens of mnemonics for even the most common disorders seen in children. Having a general idea of the overall structure of DSM-5 is helpful, but memorizing lists is of limited usefulness to the professional psychologist.

We advise psychologists to have a copy of DSM-5 itself available in every setting in which they practice. This diagnostic system cannot be used reliably or accurately without access to the diagnostic criteria and associated features for the categories. The *Desk Reference* (American Psychiatric Association, 2013a) can be a useful source of information in certain situations. This small book contains only the diagnostic criteria and *International Classification of Diseases* (ICD-9-CM, ICD-10; World Health Organization, 1977, 1992, 1993) numerical codes for the DSM-5 diagnoses; it is portable and easy to skim over, even within an evaluation session. It is important to note, however, that the *Desk Reference* omits both the text discussions and the associated features for the diagnoses. In many diagnostic decisions, especially the difficult ones, a careful consideration of the features commonly associated with various categories is essential in determining the most parsimonious but complete classification. This information must be available to examiners if their diagnostic decisions are to be informed ones. A copy of DSM-5 should be readily available in each setting in which diagnoses are formulated.

A GUIDE TO STYLISTIC CONVENTIONS IN THIS BOOK

One feature of DSM-5 that contributes slightly to its length but significantly to its lack of accessibility to many readers is the decision of its authors not to use abbreviations, even for commonly employed terms. For example, "Attention-Deficit/Hyperactivity Disorder" and "Posttraumatic Stress Disorder" are used throughout the text, whereas many publications would use these full phrases once and thereafter refer to "ADHD" and "PTSD." There are both advantages and disadvantages to this decision. The authors of DSM-5 have striven for a clarity and specificity of communication often absent from diagnostic writings. They try to say exactly what they mean, using full details rather than expecting the reader to infer what is meant. Although "ADHD" is a commonly used expression in the mental health literature and is probably familiar to almost any potential user of DSM-5, "ADHD" in the literature does not always mean the same as "Attention-Deficit/Hyperactivity Disorder" as defined within DSM-5. By stating explicitly what they mean, the authors prevent possible misunderstanding or misinterpretation. Even the use of the common DSM-IV-TR abbreviation "NOS," for "Not Otherwise Specified," has been eliminated in DSM-5, along with this designation for each disorder category. The avoidance of abbreviations can be an advantage for the occasional user of DSM-5, who does not need to refer constantly to a key to decipher terms found in the text. For these reasons, we similarly spell out the full labels of disorders in this book. The cost of this clarity, however, is a rather ponderous text, and the occasional reader can sometimes become lost in the prose.

A second stylistic convention used in this book pertains to diagnostic entities from the various editions of the DSM. Diagnostic categories from DSM-5 are given in the text with the first letter of each word capitalized, but without further elaboration: for example, "Conduct Disorder." Diagnostic categories from previous editions of the DSM are always identified according to the edition they came from: for example, "Conduct Disorder (DSM-IV-TR)" or "in DSM-IV-TR, Conduct Disorder . . . ." The exact definitions of Conduct Disorder and most other categories have changed across the different editions of the DSM. Many of these changes are subtle and possibly have had little effect on use or results. Some changes, however, have had significant effects on the populations identified with the revised categories (Tsai, 2014). Unfortunately, we often cannot know what the influence of specific wording or criterion changes have been until we are informed by subsequent research. Clearly, it appears not to be a good idea to assume much about the effects of changes in wording, symptom criteria, or frequency criteria on the application of a diagnostic category. Given this situation, within the present discussion, "Conduct Disorder" means the category as defined within DSM-5; "Conduct Disorder (DSM-IV-TR)" means the category as defined within the text revision of the fourth edition of the DSM; and "conduct disorder" or "conduct problem" has the general meaning that would be assigned to it in the psychological literature.

A third convention used herein pertains to references. References to any source other than DSM-5 (including previous versions of DSM) follow the usual style of the American Psychological Association: author, year, and page number if relevant. In references to the text of DSM-5, only a page number is given. All page-number-only references should be assumed to refer to the full text version of DSM-5 (American Psychiatric Association, 2013b).

THE SIX TYPES OF NOTES AND THEIR PURPOSES

We have used six different types of notes as "sidebars" in this book to draw certain issues to the reader's attention.

1. "Coding Notes" pertain to the use of the DSM-5 diagnostic system to classify the problems of children and adolescents. Some Coding Notes identify common errors in practice so that these can be avoided; others present supplemental material not directly pertaining to DSM-5 but relevant to the broader activity of psychodiagnosis.

2. "Application Notes" have to do with "decoding" the diagnoses given by other professionals and understanding as fully as possible the information being presented. Application Notes attempt to clarify not only the formal conventions of DSM-5 but also common practices in medical reports and other professional communications. A psychiatric diagnosis is always a summary description of an extremely complex phenomenon—the actions of another human being. In any classification effort, a certain amount of idiosyncratic information is sacrificed in order to gain the usefulness of nomothetic similarities. The challenge for the examiner is to capture the most valuable (informative) feature of a youths' presentation in the diagnoses used. The challenge for the reader is to understand as fully as possible what information is being offered by other practitioners. Application Notes attempt to aid this understanding.

3. "Professional Notes" identify "best-practice recommendations"—suggestions about diagnostic practice that are aimed at ensuring the highest level of professional psychological care for clients. Working to ensure the best service to clients, employers, and colleagues gives practicing psychologists both their best protection from personal liability and their greatest reward in personal satisfaction and professional pride. Professional Notes attempt to identify both essential elements of competent practices and exemplary levels of professional care.

4. "IDEA Notes" comment on the potential relations between DSM-5 diagnoses and classifications of eligibility for special education services under the Individuals with Disabilities Education Improvement Act (IDEA) and its amendments. Services to children are provided within the context of a number of conceptual and classification systems. Understanding the interrelations among DSM-5 and other frameworks of understanding—in this case, that of the U.S. government—can greatly enhance the utility of mental health diagnosis for practicing school and child clinical psychologists.

5. "DSM-IV-TR Notes" are offered to provide users familiar with the previous version of DSM with quick summaries of changes to each set of

diagnostic criteria. This information is purposely tucked into these notes to avoid unnecessarily weighing down the main text with overwhelming details, particularly for readers who are new to use of the DSM.

6. Finally, "Author Commentary" indicates ranting from our perspective only. One privilege of writing a book is the opportunity to voice opinions about issues of interest and concern to the audience being addressed. At the same time, responsible authorship necessitates a clear demarcation of fact from opinion (or bias). It is useful to the reader to know what the basis is for statements in this book, so we make it clear when we are presenting what DSM-5 says, what is our interpretation, what the research literature suggests, and what are our own professional opinions and experiences. We do not mind sharing our opinions with readers and hope our opinions will be given some consideration, but these comments are different from our efforts to share with you our best understanding of how to use DSM-5.

Part I

DIAGNOSTIC ISSUES AND THE USE OF DSM-5

INTRODUCTION

The initial task in learning to use DSM-5 is understanding what is involved in a mental health diagnosis. The general issues involved in psychiatric classification and the specific ways of operationalizing these issues developed by the authors of DSM-5 shape much of DSM-5's resulting taxonomy. School and child clinical psychologists usually have a general sense of the "medical model" derived from their graduate courses in abnormal behavior or developmental psychopathology, but the perspective of DSM-5 reflects the efforts of nearly a century of articulating a particular view of understanding human problems. In this perspective the clinician assumes a pivotal role. Chapter 2 explores this underlying model of the diagnostic process and the professional examiner's crucial contribution to and responsibility in applying it. Chapter 3 provides an overview of the DSM classification model and the important constructs used within this system. Chapter 4 addresses the process of learning to use DSM-5.

2

Psychiatric Diagnosis

Issues for School Psychologists

PSYCHIATRIC DIAGNOSIS AS A TASK IN SCHOOL SETTINGS

Traditional educational and psychological assessment within school settings began with psychometric measurement of cognitive abilities and academic achievement, and evolved to include evaluations of behavioral adjustment and personality. The results of these evaluations were usually communicated in descriptive narratives, with or without accompanying standard scores. Diagnostic classification was typically limited to a statement of eligibility for services (e.g., "eligible for special education") and perhaps a broad designation of the area of eligibility (e.g., "emotional disturbance"). Although most school psychologists were probably aware, on a professional level, of the publication of the landmark third edition of the DSM (DSM-III; American Psychiatric Association, 1980), it had little direct influence on their practice or daily work activities. By the time DSM-III-R was published (American Psychiatric Association, 1987), the situation had begun to change, and publications and workshops addressing the use of the DSM in school settings began to appear. The publication of DSM-IV (American Psychiatric Association, 1994) occurred in the context of broad economic, political, and social changes in the delivery of mental health services in the United States. These changes have, among many other effects, brought psychiatric diagnosis within the assigned tasks of an increasing number of school psychologists and other child-focused practitioners.

The current forces driving the increased interest in formal medical diagnosis of children's behavior and learning problems reflect the changing economic realities affecting many school districts. Despite occasional denouncements of school districts' "extravagance," the continued enactment of mandated services without accompanying mandated funding has increased the financial burden on many schools. Coincident with this situation has been the increased difficulty in obtaining school funding from traditional tax sources. The search for alternative funding sources to help relieve the expense of mandated programs has led to an interest in providing additional funding beyond special education.

One example of such an attempt is the introduction (and referral to committee) of the Mental Health in Schools Act of 2013 (H.R. 628/S. 195) as a potential amendment to the Public Health Service Act sponsored by Representative Grace Napolitano (D-California). This bill proposes to provide $200 million in competitive grants (maximum of $1 million each) to add mental health providers and services in the schools. Despite the support of 85 representatives and 65 professional organizations, including the American Counseling Association, the American Psychological Association, and the National Association of School Psychologists, this bill appears unlikely to be passed in the near future, leaving a continued, immediate need for funding. One method of such funding beyond the establishment of these types of grant-funded programs can be found by tapping into third-party reimbursement (i.e., commercial and governmental health insurance) for psychological services provided within schools.

It is at this point that the DSM enters the picture because, among the other roles played by psychiatric diagnosis, it clearly serves the primary "gatekeeping" function for insurance companies and government agencies in determining reimbursement decisions. If the school district is to gain access to potential sources of mental health service reimbursement, it is necessary for a qualified professional to determine appropriate DSM-5 classifications and corresponding ICD-9-CM (and shortly ICD-10) numerical codes for insurance review consideration. Thus, psychiatric diagnosis has increasingly become part of the task of school psychologists. The expanded attention given to diagnostic classification can be seen in a mini-series devoted to the topic in *School Psychology Review* (Power & DuPaul, 1996a). It is also reflected in the "DSM-5 and School Psychology" series of articles featured in *Communiqué*, a National Association of School Psychologists publication, that began in 2013.

PSYCHIATRIC CLASSIFICATION AND ITS ROLE IN SCHOOL SETTINGS

Psychological assessment is a broad process that encompasses many different approaches to understanding and measuring human actions and adjustment. The activities usually involved in mental health assessment differ in some important ways from the evaluation procedures traditionally used by school psychologists. First, DSM represents a categorical classification system; that is, the goal in using it is to arrive at a category or categories that most accurately reflect a youth's adjustment and functioning at this time. The purposes served by classification can include the assignment of treatment or other appropriate disposition; efficient communication with other professionals; and statistical record keeping for use in program planning, outcome research, or other application.

In addition, this classification process depends crucially upon the clinical judgment and decision making of the individual mental health professional. Psychologists need to keep in mind that DSM-5 is a document written primarily by physicians and intended primarily for the use of physicians. The working perspective in medicine is that of an individual practitioner who actively assembles relevant data, evaluates the data, arrives at working diagnoses, and acts upon the diagnoses to provide appropriate interventions. The considerable degree of authority and responsibility that the practitioner thus assumes is somewhat foreign to the practice traditions of many allied health professions. Psychology has evolved out of an academic tradition that values careful development of positions, cautious formulations of hypotheses, and consensual decisions. When one of us was a clinical psychology intern in a medical center, a supervisory psychiatrist on staff pointed out a difference he had observed in the typical oral presentations of psychology interns and psychiatry residents. The interns tended to communicate by carefully stating all the data and the rationales leading up to their final diagnostic conclusions, whereas the residents had learned to begin by stating their diagnostic impressions and, if there were questions, following these assertions up with their observations and rationales. This observation captures a valuable lesson in terms of beginning to understand the consequences of differences in professional training and traditions and in dealing with physicians. In using DSM-5, it is helpful to recognize that the judgment and decision of the professional practitioner usually serve as the basis for classification.

Although there are significant issues to be considered regarding the use of categorical diagnostic classifications with clients, especially with children, most of these are not addressed in detail here. Even to sketch the outlines of this topic would exceed the desired length of this text. Frick, Barry, and Kamphaus (2009) and Mash and Barkley (2009) present good discussions of many of the issues involved in the diagnosis and classification of psychiatric syndromes in youth. Critiques of the DSM approach in general (Kirk & Kutchins, 1992; Kutchins & Kirk, 1995) and of DSM-5 in particular (Frances, 2013; Greenberg, 2013; Wakefield, 2013) have appeared, and others will follow. This critical attention is desirable for the positive evolution of our efforts to understand and classify childhood behavior problems.

For the purposes of this book, however, it is assumed that a decision to use psychiatric diagnoses for classification purposes has already been made. Given this decision, the question becomes this: How can the DSM classification system be used to yield the most reliable, accurate, and useful results? This book is intended to help the reader become familiar with the main features of this approach to understanding and classifying emotional, behavioral, and cognitive disturbances in adjustment. In particular, we have tried to help bridge the differences in orientation and training between the school psychologists who are increasingly being called upon to use this classification system in their work settings and the practicing physicians for whom the DSM was primarily intended.

WHO CAN DIAGNOSE WITH DSM-5?

We have been asked the question in our classes for graduate students in school, clinical, and counseling psychology and in workshops for educational professionals and school administrators: Who can diagnose children using the DSM? Our first, glib and facetious, answer is "anyone who wants to," an answer intended to provoke our audience into thinking more about the question. What they are really interested in is "Who can use DSM legitimately, appropriately, legally, and ethically?" This question requires more consideration but, in our opinion, has a fairly straightforward answer as well: any professional who is competently prepared to make mental health diagnoses and is legally permitted to do so by the statues of the state in which he or she resides. In the words of DSM-5: "Clinical training and experience are needed to use DSM for determining a diagnosis" (p. 5).

There are really two issues at play in this question. First, mental health diagnosis is a professional activity with potentially serious and enduring consequences for our clients. Anyone seeking to engage in such activity has a responsibility to make sure that adequate preparation and training has been acquired to carry out this activity in the best and most responsible manner possible. Typically, graduate training in a professional human service program that includes relevant course work in human development, psychopathology, and assessment is part of the necessary training. It is likely that specific course work in using diagnostic systems such as the DSM, as well as supervised experience in practicum sites, is included in this training. Within this preparation, trainees complete readings and discussions and have opportunities to question and receive feedback on diagnostic perceptions under the supervision of an experienced professional. Second, mental health diagnosis is an activity that is regulated by state statutes in most of the United States. Part of being a professional is working to stay informed of the relevant state and federal laws that govern the performance of your services. In most states of which we are aware, mental health diagnosis is a recognized professional activity of licensed mental health professionals. Each professional in all licensed and regulated careers should ensure that he or she is practicing within his or her area of professional competence and within the proscribed boundaries of his or her profession in his or her state.

This general answer also applies to school psychologists in particular. McBride, Willis, and Dumont (2014) wrote, "We believe that a diagnosis from DSM should be within the competence of most school psychologists and that the level of training required to become proficient need not be as extensive as the level of training needed to prescribe appropriate treatments for those disabilities" (p. 427). School psychologists are well versed in developmental psychopathology and its assessment, diagnosis, and treatment. What often constrains school psychologists in diagnosing is not a lack of training but a legal prohibition of the practice by a school psychologist in a particular state. A common example is diagnosis of Attention-Deficit/Hyperactivity Disorder. Several states require diagnosis by a medical professional (e.g., a physician) for consideration of special education services for related symptoms, often in the Other Health Impairment category. It is puzzling that the trained school psychologist who is well versed in DSM-5 diagnosis and has conducted a comprehensive evaluation of the child's functioning is not permitted to provide the diagnostic label in some contexts. This example highlights the importance of understanding both the necessary qualifications for using DSM and the related legal issues. There is a difference between what a professional is competently trained to do and what the laws in a given state will allow him or her to do. It is important to be aware that these are two separate but related issues. It is easy to fuse our understanding of the law and local customs with our understanding of our professional capabilities. In the case of providing DSM diagnoses, these two issues are not in agreement as practiced in some states. It is unfortunate that many state laws have prevented the cost-effective use of school psychologists' expertise to streamline these processes.

DEVELOPMENTAL CONSIDERATIONS IN DIAGNOSING CHILDREN AND ADOLESCENTS

Although, as we have stated previously, space considerations preclude a detailed debate of the merits and demerits of a categorical diagnostic system such as DSM-5, most commentators agree that the application of such a system to children and adolescents is especially challenging. In this section, we discuss some of the developmental features that must be taken into consideration in the psychiatric diagnosis of children and adolescents.

A typical adult client presents himself or herself to a mental health professional and reports the concerns that have led him or her to seek services—for instance, sadness and crying spells, discouraging marital conflicts, or questions about career direction. The most commonly used assessment tool/approach is the clinical interview. Based on the verbal information reported by the adult client, the professional arrives at an assessment (which may include a DSM diagnosis), proposes a treatment plan, and makes a disposition of the case. Often implicit in this exchange are the assumptions that the client's report of his or her circumstances is largely accurate; that the client's personality and cognitive functioning are relatively stable over time; and that (within certain ethical boundaries) the agenda of therapy is largely shaped by the client's wishes and goals. These modal features of work with adults influence many aspects of service provision, including the practices leading to diagnosis.

Professionals working primarily with children and adolescents deal routinely with quite different initial characteristics. Young persons almost never refer themselves for treatment or other psychological services; adult caretakers (parents, teachers, other concerned adults) refer them because they become concerned about their adjustment, functioning, progress, or happiness. A basic truism is that what children and adolescents may worry about most may not be what concerns their caretakers most. For instance, fears of animals constitute the most common extreme anxiety reactions of children, yet fears of animals are not the most commonly seen fears in professional practice with children. Fears of school are not frequent among children's anxiety problems; however, historically "school phobia" has been one of the most commonly seen and investigated childhood fears in clinical circumstances (Miller, Barrett, & Hampe, 1974). This disparity illustrates one of the most important factors in assessing child and adolescent psychopathology: Adults refer young children because of behavior that causes the adults concern. This prerequisite has profound implications for what problems are noticed, are studied, become better understood, and evolve into recognized diagnostic entries.

Children and adolescents also appear to be more influenced by environmental variables than adults; their behavior is more situationally specific. Many aspects of young persons' adjustment and functioning, including their problems, are more fluid and evolving than is the case for most adults. This plasticity creates problems for categorical classification systems, in which it is assumed that the classified things or individuals remain relatively constant unless they are deliberately changed. This greater responsiveness to environmental contingencies also means that a greater degree of attention must be devoted to evaluating situational characteristics and variables in arriving at an understanding or diagnosis of young people's problems. For instance, the requirement in DSM-5 of basing a diagnosis of Attention-Deficit/Hyperactivity Disorder upon manifestation of symptoms in at least two settings greatly affects the identified population and its modal characteristics. Requiring cross-situational manifestation (pervasive Attention-Deficit/Hyperactivity Disorder) reduces the number of children identified as having Attention-Deficit/Hyperactivity Disorder, may reduce false-positive diagnoses, may increase false-negative diagnoses, and probably leads to a focus on more severely disturbed children—thereby altering the modal features of a child diagnosed with Attention-Deficit/Hyperactivity Disorder.

In addition to the need to attend to environmental features, the language and cognitive differences between youth and adults must be taken into consideration. A primary reliance on verbal reports in the context of a clinical interview is often seen as a much less acceptable source of data for evaluating children and adolescents than for evaluating adults. For example, clinically depressed children, especially preschool and early primary school children, may not report themselves to be sad. They may report physical concerns or vague complaints of "not feeling well." Their nonverbal behavior may prompt others to express concerns about their well-being. They may show, but not necessarily report, a decrease in activities they previously enjoyed. In the words of one of our students, children tend to "walk the walk" of depression rather than "talk the talk." Interviews with parents and other collateral informants, behavior rating scales, naturalistic observations, and formal psychological testing all play a relatively more important role in the assessment of children and adolescents than in that of adults. These differences have implications for the use of DSM-5 with children and adolescents and bring into focus some of the recurrent dissatisfactions with the DSM system. In this book, we try to point out occasions in which additional sources of information can be especially useful in applying DSM-5 classifications to the evaluation of young people.

3

An Overview of the DSM-5 Diagnostic System

BASIC DEFINITIONS OF MENTAL DISORDERS AND OTHER CONDITIONS

DSM-5 is concerned with classifying mental disorders. There are several considerations to take into account in order to understand exactly what this statement means. The first issue centers on the definition of "mental disorder"—that is, the standards by which professionals determine whether a diagnosable condition is present. One also must take into account the relation between mental disorders and other phenomena of interest—especially the observable characteristics of individuals, their self-reports, and theories about the cause and prevention of mental disorders. Finally, it is important to recognize and remember that DSM-5 is a categorical (qualitative) classification system. Despite efforts to consider dimensional (quantitative) models of behavioral phenomena, DSM-5 is explicitly and fundamentally a categorical system. It provides rules for establishing whether a given pattern of behavior does or does not meet criteria for inclusion in an identified group. A major advantage of categorical classification is the ease with which diagnoses inform dispositional actions such as treatment, placement, and referral. One of the frequently discussed "pros" of mental health diagnosis is the facilitation of appropriate treatment efforts. If we have a valid and reliable classification scheme and empirically supported treatments, the diagnoses become vehicles to link clients with the most helpful interventions.

DSM-5 offers a definition of "Mental Disorder," as did DSM-IV-TR, DSM-IV, DSM-III-R, and DSM-III. There are only minor differences among the definitions provided in these editions. Since DSM-III, the cognitive and behavioral disorders classified by DSM-5 as Mental Disorders have been identified by means of one or both of two defining characteristics: significant personal distress in the individual affected and/or significant adaptive failure. The additional criteria discussed can be viewed as various special cases of the second criterion. Each and every time the term "disorder" is used in DSM-5 in the context of a mental, emotional, or behavioral problem, the meaning is that, in addition to any other specific criteria that are met, one or both of these two general criteria are also met. All Mental Disorders, by definition, meet this basic DSM-5 criterion: "A mental disorder is a syndrome characterized by clinically significant disturbance in an individual's cognition, emotion regulation, or behavior that reflects a dysfunction in the psychological, biological, or developmental processes underlying mental functioning" (p. 20).

The discussion in the text goes on to exclude expectable or culturally approved responses to a particular event (such as the death of a loved one); to require that the problem be associated with significant distress or disability in social, occupational, or other important functions (regardless of what its original cause may have been); and to address the boundaries of social deviance and mental disorder: "Socially deviant behavior (e.g., political, religious, or sexual) and conflicts that are primarily between the individual and society are not mental disorders unless the deviance or conflict results from dysfunction in the individual, as described above" (p. 20). A distinct feature of the DSM system has been the formal declaration (since DSM-III) that the classification is not a classification of people but rather of the disorders that people experience.

The idea of a disorder, mental or otherwise, involves a perception of an enduring group of associated characteristics. The basic elements are objective data about an individual and his or her (subjective) self-reports. A "sign" is some observable (measurable), objective characteristic of the person. For example, increased heart rate, perspiration, and behavioral avoidance when confronted with a feared object are several signs of anxiety in a client. A "symptom" refers to the subjective report of the person. The client's statements that he or she is fearful, is nervous, and wishes to get away from the feared situation are all symptoms of anxiety. The observation or statistical determination that a number of signs and symptoms may go together forms the basis of identification of syndromes. "Syndromes" are patterns of covariation between signs and symptoms. There is a trend toward increased consistency among authors in their use of these three terms. Signs, symptoms, and syndromes provide the basic elements of many modern conceptualizations of emotional and behavioral problems, including the DSM.

The Criterion A requirements of most of the DSM-5 diagnoses identify the relevant syndrome for each diagnosis. A syndrome is what many students tend to think of as the defining feature of a Mental Disorder, but there are usually other elements just as important and essential. There may also be the inclusion of requirements of duration. Some syndromes are identified as events. The discussion of "panic attack," which is used as the core element of several anxiety disorder definitions, involves several signs and symptoms occurring together. This cluster is a classic presentation of a syndrome. The discussion of mood disorders illustrates the use of time requirements. A major depressive syndrome is specified with the additional requirement that the cluster of symptoms and signs have occurred for a minimum of 2 weeks: This period is identified as a "depressive episode." There may also be exclusion criteria—identification of other problems (Mental Disorders or General Medical Conditions) that would preclude a given diagnosis from being made if they were present.

A disorder is, then, identified as a syndrome that meets certain additional criteria. In DSM-5, the requirements for all disorders are evidence of significant personal distress, functional impairment, or contribution to personal risk of loss (see the basic definition of "Mental Disorder" given earlier). One change from DSM-III-R to DSM-IV that has been maintained in DSM-5 is the overt inclusion of these requirements in most of the diagnostic criterion sets. This repetition does not represent any conceptual change—the requirement was there as early as DSM-III—but these fundamental requirements were not repeated over and over before DSM-IV. The decision to add them (as several lines of text) to most DSM-5 criterion sets is an attempt to decrease overdiagnosis of subclinical problems by reminding examiners that all Mental Disorders not only must meet the specific criteria for a particular type of behavioral or emotional problem but must also show the characteristics that define psychopathology for DSM-5. The fundamental task of the examiner in using DSM-5 is to decide whether the human difficulties he or she is presented with can be reasonably conceptualized as Mental Disorders within the DSM system.

An "illness" is a disorder with known etiology and pathophysiology; that is, a full understanding exists of the causes and mechanisms of the problems. Few of the disorders defined in DSM-5 are close to the point where they might be conceptualized as illnesses. Indeed, some would maintain that most human behavioral enactments cannot be reasonably considered as illnesses with "illness" so defined. Nevertheless, recent developments in the study of several mental disorders raise intriguing possibilities that at least a few may ultimately be understood in this form. This type of understanding is often one of the goals of medical research, and the expansion of our knowledge about behavioral and emotional problems may require a fundamental reorganization of our view of some of these problems. Some research on autism, for instance, suggests that this pattern of behavior and maladjustment may be a final common pathway of several etiological processes, some of which may ultimately be well conceptualized as illnesses. These topics, however, are far beyond the scope of this book, which focuses on the application of the current DSM diagnostic system.

Mental Disorders are not the only problems classified in DSM-5. Various human relationship difficulties and other conditions that cause upset in adjustment and functioning are considered because these problems are frequently the focus of clinical attention. Beginning on page 715, these "Other Conditions That May Be a Focus of Clinical Attention" provide for the specification of a wide range of problematic circumstances in the lives of individuals being evaluated. Many of these other conditions may be among the problems most frequently seen by the practicing psychologist or counselor. These problems are viewed as important within DSM-5, and there are provisions for coding them, but they are not Mental Disorders within the meaning of that term in DSM-5. These problems are not Mental Disorders because they do not meet the basic requirements for a Mental Disorder—significant distress, functional impairment, and/or special risk. The defining aspect of these other conditions is that, in the judgment of the examiner, they warrant clinical attention. An easy operationalization of this idea is the development of a treatment plan to address one of these other conditions or inclusion of the problem as a specific treatment target in the intervention plan for a related Mental Disorder. Identification of one or more other conditions in a youth's diagnosis does not require such formal justification, but there is the clear implication that these are serious difficulties for the young person and that they justify some attention.

The consideration that a problem is severe enough to be a focus of treatment is a general criterion used in identifying Other Conditions That May Be a Focus of Clinical Attention, as well as in deciding at the time whether to make an additional, separate diagnosis of an associated symptom area when the youth has an identified Mental Disorder. For instance, a Sleep Disorder would not normally be diagnosed in a teenager with Major Depressive Disorder because sleep problems are symptoms of depression; however, if the sleep disturbance is judged to be a critical treatment focus, an independent diagnosis can be made. If the adolescent were referred to a sleep disorder specialist for evaluation and treatment, the sleep disorder would become the primary diagnosis for that provider and the depressive disorder secondary.

In addition to Other Conditions That May Be a Focus of Clinical Attention, various psychological, social, and medical characteristics of a child or adolescent may be classified within DSM-5 and do not constitute Mental Disorders. Before these are described, it is necessary to take a look at the overall organization of classification in DSM-5.

REMOVAL OF THE MULTIAXIAL SYSTEM OF CLASSIFICATION

Beginning with DSM-III in 1980, the American Psychiatric Association's diagnostic system was structured around five "axes" or categories of information (see Table 3.1). Multiaxial approaches to diagnosis were recommended as a means of ensuring a more complete assessment of each client as a total person—that is, of encouraging a review of several aspects of adjustment and functioning, rather than just symptoms. Each of the two subsequent revisions of the DSM saw slight modifications of the axes' content, but the basic structure was left intact. The term "axis" may be somewhat misleading for the reader if it is taken to imply a dimensional or

TABLE 3.1. DSM-IV-TR Multiaxial Assessment

Axis I: Clinical Disorders and Other Conditions That May Be a Focus of Clinical Attention

Most diagnoses in the basic body of DSM-IV were made on Axis I. These were the acute clinical conditions that usually brought a client to an examiner's attention. Most Axis I disorders are viewed as afflictions that have developed in a client's life at some point ("onset"); troubled the client over some period of time ("course"); and eventually end ("in remission").

Other Conditions That May Be a Focus of Clinical Attention (often called "V codes") were also coded on Axis I. These were issues that could affect the adjustment of a child or the course or prognosis of a disorder, but they were not Mental Disorders in the sense of DSM-IV. Some examples were Physical Child Abuse, Marital Conflict, and Borderline Intellectual Functioning; all were important issues that could have serious influences on the adjustment of a youth, but they were not considered Mental Disorders.

Axis II: Mental Retardation; Personality Disorders

Axis II took several forms over the DSM editions of III, III-R, and IV. In DSM-IV-TR only Mental Retardation (Intellectual Disability in DSM-5) and Personality Disorders were coded on Axis II. Personality traits and ego defenses could be noted (although these were not coded with ICD designations).

Axis III: General Medical Conditions

Medical diagnoses were coded, and other relevant health information could be noted.

Axis IV: Psychosocial and Environmental Problems

Additional contextual variables for consideration, such as poverty, limited access to medical care, sexual abuse, and juvenile court involvement, were addressed on Axis IV.

Axis V: Global Assessment of Functioning (GAF)

The examiner made a rating of the client's overall adjustment, considering both symptoms and the individual's social and occupational/school functioning.

continuous variable. Only one of the axes—Axis V, Global Assessment of Functioning (GAF)—constitutes a continuous scale. The other axes involve various categorical classifications of different types of information: acute clinical problems, enduring characteristics of the individual, medical conditions, and environmental stressors.

DSM-5 removes the multiaxial approach to assessment. (See Author Commentary: A Lament for the Demise of the Multiaxial System on the next page.) All mental health diagnoses, medical diagnoses, and other conditions that are the focus of clinical attention are listed together. Unless otherwise specified, the reader will presume that the first diagnosis given is the primary diagnosis (the reason that the youth is being seen or the first problem to be focused on in treatment). Several factors may have contributed to the demise of the multiaxial system. One was dissatisfaction with the differentiation of mental health diagnoses and other medical conditions. There was also difficulty with giving a clear, conceptual definition to the distinction between Axis I and Axis II. The original intent in the construction of Axis II was to ensure that "consideration is given to the possible presence of disorders that are frequently overlooked when attention is directed to the more florid Axis I disorder" (American Psychiatric Association, 1980, p. 23). Discussions focused on more enduring versus acute problems, but it was difficult to draw a clear conceptual definition. Several disorders migrated between Axis I and Axis II over the next several iterations. Yet another dissatisfaction may have been difficulty with the reliability of the GAF ratings for Axis V. Several other considerations may have played a role in this change. The issues are discussed briefly in DSM-5 (p. 16). Regardless of the reasons, this change marks a fundamental difference in organization and conceptualization between DSM-5 and the previous four editions (i.e., DSM-III, DSM-III-R, DSM-IV, DSM-IV-TR).

In the current edition, diagnoses are listed either by primacy of clinical need or reason for seeking treatment. Within most DSM-5 diagnostic categories, diagnoses are further differentiated by the use of "subtypes or presentations" and "specifiers." *Subtypes* are "mutually exclusive and jointly exhaustive" patterns of phenomenological characteristics (p. 21). For example, Conduct Disorder has three subtypes based on the age of onset of problems: Childhood-Onset Type, Adolescent-Onset Type, and Unspecified Onset. *Specifiers* are "not intended to be mutually exclusive or jointly exhaustive," but instead "provide an opportunity to define a more homogeneous subgrouping of individuals" within a diagnostic category (pp. 21–22). In a diagnosis of Stereotypic Movement Disorder, for instance, several specifiers are available: With Self-Injurious Behavior, Without Self-Injurious Behavior; Associated with a Known Medical or Genetic Condition, Neurodevelopmental Disorder, or Environmental Factor; and Mild, Moderate, and Severe degrees of severity. *Distinctive Feature specifiers*

Author Commentary. A Lament for the Demise of the Multiaxial System

A major innovation in the third edition of the DSM was the introduction of a "multiaxial" system of classification. Mental health diagnoses were to be more than a listing of codified syndromes and disorders; they were to be a deliberate effort to communicate as much useful information about the patient as possible. The mechanism adopted to achieve this end was elaborating diagnoses into five axes to ensure economically capturing as many data as possible. Axis I encompassed the clinical syndromes and other conditions that might be the focus of clinical attention (with what were called the "V codes" because, in the then-current ICD-9 system, clinical focuses of attention that were not mental disorders usually were designated with an initial V and then a numeric code). Axis II was for identifying more chronic or enduring conditions that might not be fully considered in the context of the dramatic and florid Axis I conditions. A major problem was defining Axis II and what should be on Axis II; these questions were never satisfactorily answered. Personality disorders (and personality traits) were always on Axis II; autism was on Axis I in DSM-III and then moved to Axis II in III-R and then back to Axis I in DSM-IV; learning disabilities were on Axis II in DSM-III and DSM-III-R, and then moved to Axis I in DSM-IV. Axis III was used for medical and physiological conditions. Axis IV included environmental and psychosocial conditions that affected the expression, prognosis, or response to treatment of Axis I or Axis II conditions. Axis V was the Global Assessment of Functioning (GAF) scale.

Let us just admit from the beginning that there were multiple specific problems with this system: the difficulty of differentiating Axis I and Axis II, the philosophical issue of whether mental disorders and medical disorders were really the same or different, the inadequate attention given to developing Axis IV, the lack of reliability of Axis V ratings, the heterogeneity of Axis V rating factors (some specific actions, such as suicide attempts, would drive rating powerfully), and still other issues. Indeed, there were problems with the multiaxial system, but the goal of directing us to consider as broadly as possible the diverse and interwoven influences on clinical expression was worthwhile and deserved continuing efforts to address these problems. Instead, the authors of DSM-5 have given up on the project. Mental health diagnoses are going to be just like other medical diagnoses (a cynic might suspect that this is the most powerful motivation for this change): a single ICD code attached to a categorical conceptualization of disordered human behavior. Gone is the effort to include as much of the full human condition as possible in our representation of our clients' current challenging situations. The change has been made. The multiaxial system is gone. Our students will say: "It is what it is." In this case, it is just sad. We are capable of better.

may indicate potentially clinically relevant distinctions (e.g., With Good Insight; With Mixed Features; With Impairment in Written Expression). *Course specifiers* indicate the current status of the disorder (e.g., "In Partial Remission," "In Full Remission"). Usually DSM-5 diagnoses are assumed to reflect the current status of the client. Previous diagnoses that are not currently fully present may be noted with qualification (e.g., "In Partial Remission," "In Full Remission"). *Severity specifiers* indicate the examiner's judgment of the "intensity, frequency, duration, symptom count, or other severity indicator of a disorder" (p. 22).

Severity specifiers are a frequently employed class of specifiers in DSM-5. The specifiers Mild, Moderate, and Severe may be used when a case meets full criteria for most diagnoses; for several diagnoses, explicit criteria for the specifiers are provided. Both frequency and qualitative features are considered in choosing a severity specifier. The designation Mild is used when the manifest symptoms only just meet the diagnostic criteria requirements for the category. Severe usually means that many more symptoms than the minimum necessary for diagnosis can be documented. Moderate is used to qualify cases with an intermediate frequency of symptoms between Mild and Severe. The assignment of a severity specifier, however, is complicated by the additional consideration of the intensity and/or functional influence of symptoms.

As an illustration, consider Conduct Disorder again. This diagnosis requires the presence of at least three of 15 symptoms during the preceding year. When the criteria for the disorder are met, we usually specify the Conduct Disorder diagnosis of a child with three or four symptoms as Mild, as Severe for a child with 12 or more symptoms, and as Moderate somewhere in between these extremes. The assignment of Mild requires only the necessary three symptoms *and* only minor harm to others, whereas the assignment of Severe requires many conduct problems beyond the three needed for criteria *or* "considerable harm to others." That is, a child who only met three or four of the symptoms of Conduct Disorder but whose actions severely injured other children on repeated occasions could justifiably be classified as having "severe" Conduct Disorder. A child who often bullies other children at school, initiates frequent fights on a regular basis, and has violently beaten another child with a baseball bat will probably be diagnosed as having Conduct Disorder, Severe, on the basis of the harm caused in the one attack with a weapon. Our experience suggests that intra- and interrater reliability rates in the use of severity specifiers are probably significantly lower than agreement on the basic diagnosis. Although some useful information can be captured and conveyed with these qualifiers, the reader should appreciate the greater degree of subjectivity involved in these determinations than in the basic diagnosis.

Course specifiers, another group of specifiers, contrast a client's present status with his or her previous mental health history. In general, In Partial Remission means that full criteria were previously met but that only some of the original symptoms presently remain. In Full Remission means that there is currently a complete absence of symptoms but that in the examiner's judgment it is clinically relevant to note the client's adjustment history. There is no absolute demarcation between In Full Remission and Recovered (when the disorder would no longer be noted). Even when a client is judged to be recovered, the prior history of a disorder can be noted if the examiner believes that this information has value for an understanding of the case. As an example, the literature on reading problems suggests that there may often be a history of developmental articulation problems that have been completely resolved in the backgrounds of poor readers. A diagnosis for such a child might be as follows:

Specific Learning Disorder, with impairment in reading
Prior History of Speech Sound Disorder (recovered)

or

Specific Learning Disorder, with impairment in reading
Speech Sound Disorder, In Full Remission

The distinction between these two is left up to the examiner, but relevant variables may include the age of the child, the amount of time that has elapsed since criteria for the Speech Sound Disorder were met, and where on the spectrum of "within normal limits" the child's current articulation falls.

For several disorders and their associated syndromes (Manic Episode, Major Depressive Episode, Substance Dependence), there are specific criteria for the qualifiers In Partial Remission and In Full Remission. For the Substance Dependence disorders, as an example, the course specifiers are Early Full Remission, Early Partial Remission, Sustained Full Remission, and Sustained Partial Remission. The qualifier Sustained Full Remission is used if there have been no symptoms of Substance Dependence or

Coding Note. Implementation of ICD-10

The DSM-5 lists alphanumeric codes for each disorder. These codes were established by the World Health Organization in the *International Classification of Diseases*. The DSM-5 lists both the codes for the 9th revision and the 10th revision of the ICD because the United States has not yet implemented clinical use of the 10th revision even though it was published in 1992. Implementation of the 10th revision was scheduled for fall 2014, but this date was delayed for a year, with a revised implementation date of October 1, 2015. When implemented in the United States, ICD-10 will be referenced as ICD-10-CM, meaning the clinical modification of the 10th revision of the ICD adopted in the United States. See Goodheart (2014) for further discussion and references on this topic.

Substance Abuse for 12 months or longer. These course specifiers, however, are precluded by either of two additional specifiers: On Agonist Therapy or In a Controlled Environment.

Also included in the manual are behavior and situational problems that justify professional involvement but do not fall within the DSM-5 definition of a Mental Disorder. As noted earlier, the class of Other Conditions That May Be a Focus of Clinical Attention greatly expands the range of application of DSM-5. Often still referred to as "V codes," although they no longer all begin with the letter V in ICD-9-CM and none will in ICD-10-CM, these conditions allow the examiner to address real concerns in the lives of many youth—problems such as family conflict, physical or sexual abuse, unemployment, and identity issues. This section has been significantly expanded in DSM-5, with a number of new categories available that were not present previously. It is important for child clinical and school psychologists to be familiar with this section of DSM-5. (For a brief discussion of the implementation of ICD codes in the United States as they relate to clinical practice, see the previous Coding Note.)

For most nonmedically trained examiners, the use of medical diagnoses is one of the most problematic aspects of applying DSM-5. Yet the relevance of many medical conditions to the understanding of an increasing number of childhood disorders can hardly be denied. Skodol (1989) discussed the use of Axis III (General Medical Conditions) in DSM-IV by nonmedical mental health professionals and offered the opinion that notation on Axis III does not indicate that a particular diagnosis is being made by the person recording the multiaxial evaluation. He suggested that nonmedical clinicians may wish to indicate the sources of their information on Axis III. This simple convention can reduce the anxiety of most examiners about including a medical diagnosis in their evaluation and prevent any professional concerns about nonphysicians diagnosing a medical illness (see the following Professional Note). Although the multiaxial system has been removed in DSM-5, this practice of providing medical information along with the source of this information within a case conceptualization and diagnosis is recommended.

PRECEDENCE OF DIAGNOSES: DIAGNOSTIC CONVENTIONS, HIERARCHIES, AND MULTIPLE DIAGNOSES

In general, DSM-5 actively encourages multiple diagnoses, so that the salient problems experienced by a client can be fully described. This comprehensive inclusion is one of the clearest contrasts between the approach taken to classification by the DSM committee and that taken by the authors of the *International Classification of Diseases* (ICD). The philosophy of

Professional Note. The Use of Medical Diagnoses by the Nonphysician

We recommend as best practice that the school psychologist or other nonmedical professional indicate the sources of all medical information or determinations, as shown in these examples:

> Mother reported that child has juvenile-onset diabetes.
> Genetic karyotype indicates trisomy 21.
> Seizure disorder diagnosed by child's pediatrician, James Lee, MD.

ICD-9 (World Health Organization, 1977) appeared to encourage as much parsimony as possible in diagnosis. This approach may change with the implementation of ICD-10 in the United States, which appears to accept the possibility of a client needing the designation of multiple diagnoses (World Health Organization, 1992, 1993). As mentioned, the DSM philosophy from DSM-III onward has been to encourage multiple diagnoses. A consequence of this approach is that individual cases typically receive more than one diagnosis. The confusion caused by diagnostic proliferation has been a criticism of the DSM. In contrast to previous editions of the DSM, most rules of diagnostic precedence (see DSM-IV-TR, pp. 6–7, and Fauman, 1994) no longer apply in DSM-5. In DSM-5 even more emphasis is placed on the examiner to generate the best conceptualization of the case and to determine diagnostic primacy.

Some diagnostic possibilities, however, continue to take precedence over others. As with DSM-IV, any manifestation of a clear history of manic or hypomanic episode forever leads to a diagnosis of a Bipolar Disorder rather than a Depressive Disorder. The determination of when there has, in fact, been a previous manic or hypomanic episode can be a challenge for the examiner, especially because being seen by others or by oneself as "bipolar" seems to be somewhat common in some populations. Unfortunately, for many this term appears to have become a catch phrase for having problems with temper or impulse control (e.g., "I snapped out") rather than referring to enduring mood shifts. Even the use of symptom rating scales, such as the Child Mania Rating Scale, usually need to be carefully followed up with questioning to determine the exact behaviors informants are reporting. The examiner should carefully read the criteria for Manic Episode, Hypomanic Episode, and Major Depressive Episode and the diagnostic criteria for Persistent Depressive Disorder (Dysthymia) and review them often. Another explicit rule of precedence is between Conduct

Disorder and Antisocial Personality Disorder in adults (a diagnosis of Antisocial Personality Disorder cannot be made prior to age 18). In an adult, if criteria for Antisocial Personality Disorder are met, this diagnosis takes precedence over a diagnosis of Conduct Disorder.

A general rule of diagnostic formulation throughout DSM-5 is that when any problem is considered to be a manifestation of a known biological illness or chemical influence, these influences take precedence in diagnosis. The majority of the diagnostic criterion sets include criteria that make this clear: "not attributable to the physiological effects of a substance" "or another medical condition." This practice continues the pattern of DSM-IV: It included the statement " . . . is not due to the direct physiological effects of a substance (e.g., a drug of abuse, or a medication) or a general medical condition." This repetition tells the reader that these conditions preempt the diagnosis of other Mental Disorders. Symptoms of severe and sustained depression that arise as a consequence of alcohol abuse, for instance, should not be diagnosed as Major Depressive Disorder but as Alcohol-Induced Depressive Disorder.

The third general directive pertains to circumstances in which a given clinical situation could possibly be accounted for by two different diagnoses. In such circumstances the examiner must review all the data available and make a determination as to which diagnosis best represents a client's situation. The text phrase is used to alert the reader to possible alternative conceptualizations: It reads, " . . . is not better explained by . . . " in the diagnostic criteria set.

CHILD AND ADOLESCENT MENTAL HEALTH AND DSM-5

Our understanding of mental health problems in children and adolescents lags behind the level of knowledge that has been achieved with adults. Several factors have contributed to this disparity, and some of these continue to operate. For many decades, emotional and behavioral problems in young people were treated solely as juvenile extensions of the difficulties seen in adults, with little or no appreciation of the unique developmental features of childhood and adolescence that can affect the forms psychopathology takes. The research methods necessitated by these developmental features (e.g., large-scale, longitudinal studies and naturalistic observation methodologies) are often time-consuming, labor-intensive, and expensive—factors that have further slowed progress. For research involving some degree of risk (e.g., intervention studies or intensive assessment investigations), there is an understandable caution about conducting research on young people, but this avoidance of risk also has the cost of slowing our learning. Finally, there is a real possibility that psychopathology in the rapidly changing child or adolescent is to some degree a different phenomenon from that seen in the more consistently behaving adult. The behaviors of children and adolescents change as they learn, grow, and develop. Clearly, some patterns of psychopathology change over time, but possibly the very construct of mental disorder in young people refers to more fluid and less consistent manifestations than those seen in adults, who generally have established life routines.

For the practicing school psychologist or other psychologist working with children, one of the most important aspects in learning to use DSM-5 accurately is to recognize that there is no "child section" of DSM-5, nor are there any "child diagnoses." The clear position of the American Psychiatric Association from DSM-III through DSM-III-R to DSM-IV to DSM-5 has been that basic mental health phenomena are essentially the same, regardless of age or developmental stage. For example, the manifestation and experience of severe depression are seen as similar in children, in adolescents, in adults, and in geriatric populations. There is some recognition of age-associated features, but these are seen as minor variations on the major themes. Similarly, there is no separate discussion of "Childhood Schizophrenia" as a separate taxonomic category from Schizophrenia in adults. The core symptoms of the disorder labeled Schizophrenia are seen as basically the same, regardless of an individual's age; developmental features provide some secondary elaborations of these manifestations but do not change the essential equation. One consequence of this formulation is that the school psychologist must be just as familiar with the entire text of DSM-5 as the psychologist who usually sees adult or geriatric populations.

Although there is no child section or chapter from which the school psychologist can safely assume that all his or her diagnostic decisions will originate DSM-5 has adopted a general developmental organization to the order of presentation of chapters and topics. Major problem areas that usually manifest earlier in the life of an individual are addressed, in general, earlier in the text. The first chapter of diagnostic categories, Neurodevelopmental Disorders, focuses on diagnoses usually first made in early life (e.g., Intellectual Disabilities, Attention-Deficit/Hyperactivity Disorder). However, this developmental ordering pertains to the broad area and not to specific diagnoses. Elimination Disorders, for instance, are considered much later in the text, as are Disruptive, Impulse-Control, and Conduct Disorders. The clinical child specialist will need to be familiar with the entire text of DSM-5 to appropriately use this system.

A positive change with DSM-5 has been much greater attention given to developmental considerations. The topic of how diagnostic presentations may change over the lifespan is discussed in much greater detail for most categories. The course (pattern of onset, duration, pattern of exacerbation and remission) of a problem set is fundamental to the definition of most DSM-5 diagnoses (e.g., Schizophrenia), but previous editions gave less attention to how the symptom picture could differ in child, adolescent, adult, and older-age populations.

4

Learning to Use DSM-5

CATEGORICAL CLASSIFICATION

The most important information for each diagnosis in DSM-5 is found in the sentence that begins: "The essential feature(s) of [Name of Disorder or Class of Disorders] is . . . " under the heading "Diagnostic Features." This statement provides the conceptual foundation for each diagnosis. The diagnostic criteria for each specific diagnosis (or group of diagnoses) document different patterns of manifestation *within the context identified by the essential feature*. The essential feature, then, is like a street address of a particular friend, but before finding it, the examiner needs to be sure that he or she is in the right "city." This concept is illustrated by the last two diagnoses given in most sections and chapters: Other Specified and Unspecified Disorder options. These two diagnostic options replace the DSM-IV designation "Not Otherwise Specified" with the choice either to specify why the diagnostic criteria for a class of disorders are not met but still warrant clinical attention and diagnosis or to omit information about which criteria were not met (i.e., Unspecified Disorder). These two options list no diagnostic criteria and are sometimes disparagingly described as a "blank check" that evaluators can use to give any diagnosis that they please without being bothered by the restrictions of diagnostic criteria. This criticism is not a valid view of the application of an Other Specified/Unspecified diagnosis. Such a diagnosis is properly applied when an evaluator has concluded that the particular case is best understood as an instance of the general problem area identified—that is, that a youth's problems are best captured within a group of difficulties sharing an essential feature.

Here is an illustration of this difference in orientation. Within the "Neurodevelopmental Disorders" chapter is the section on Attention-Deficit/Hyperactivity Disorder; these disorders include the category Attention-Deficit/Hyperactivity Disorder and the categories of Other Specified Attention-Deficit/Hyperactivity Disorder and Unspecified Attention-Deficit/Hyperactivity Disorder. This section begins as follows: "The essential feature of attention-deficit/hyperactivity disorder is a persistent pattern of inattention and/or hyperactivity–impulsivity that interferes with functioning or development" (p. 61). The basic Attention-Deficit/Hyperactivity Disorder category contains three presentations based on various combinations of symptoms from the Attention-Deficit/Hyperactivity Disorder criteria set. The Other Specified and Unspecified Attention-Deficit/Hyperactivity Disorder categories are one paragraph in length and begin with the statement "This category applies to presentations in which symptoms characteristic of attention-deficit/hyperactivity disorder that cause clinically significant distress or impairment in social, occupational or other important areas of functioning predominate but do not meet the full criteria for attention-deficit/hyperactivity disorder or any of the disorders in the neurodevelopmental disorders diagnostic class" (p. 65). The examiner is free to use the Other Specified or Unspecified Attention-Deficit/Hyperactivity Disorder categories to diagnose children (or adults) who do not meet the various criteria for Attention-Deficit/Hyperactivity Disorder. The expectation in allowing this latitude is that the problematic pattern of behavior and adjustment being considered *does* include the essential feature of the category being considered and that one of these diagnoses is the best organizing principle for the available data. The Other Specified/Unspecified options give the evaluator a significant degree of freedom, but they also place a significant burden on him or her to use the system in a responsible and appropriate manner. The authors of DSM-5 make the point that the classification system is not intended to be applied in a rigid, cookbook manner that reduces the professional to a technician; they note that the diagnostic criteria are provided as "guidelines for making diagnoses, and their use should be informed by clinical judgment" (p. 21). This point is directly relevant to the use of the Other Specified/Unspecified diagnoses.

DIFFERENTIAL DIAGNOSIS

The primary task of the school psychologist or other professional examiner using DSM-5 to diagnose a child or adolescent is to determine which category or categories best capture the nature of the young person's current problems in adjustment and functioning. The presenting concerns that bring the youth to the examiner's attention could potentially be signs of several different patterns of maladjustment. For instance, a teacher's report that a child exhibits aggressive behavior during recess and class changes might indicate an adjustment disorder, a mood disorder, a conduct disorder, or some other diagnosis. The collection of additional data regarding the child, the child's history of problems, and his or her concomitant difficulties allow a rational choice to be made among the various diagnostic possibilities. "Ruling in" (identifying) or "ruling out" (excluding from consideration; see the following Application Note) different categories is known as the process of "differential diagnosis." For most major diagnoses, the text of DSM-5 identifies which alternative conceptualizations are most likely to be considered, and it attempts to highlight relevant differences.

A new user of DSM-5 may be somewhat overwhelmed by these sections of the manual; to many of us, it initially appears that "everything is a differential diagnosis for everything." With only a little experience, however, certain underlying relations become more familiar, and the process of differential diagnosis becomes more selective. First (2014) offers decision trees for 29 disturbances in functioning, many of which are relevant to children and adolescents. These decision trees, in addition to guiding

Application Note. "Rule Out"

The phrase "rule out" does not appear in DSM-5 and is not part of the vocabulary of the DSM. However, it is a common expression in psychiatric diagnosis and is often seen in reports, especially from professionals with medical training or experience in medical settings. There is often some confusion among nonphysicians as to the meaning of this expression. "Rule out" is typically used to identify an alternative diagnosis that is being actively considered but for which sufficient data have not yet been obtained. For instance, the diagnostic statement "Oppositional Defiant Disorder, rule out Conduct Disorder," suggests that the examiner has concluded there is definitely a problem with compliance with authority and rule following in at least one setting and that the more serious problem of Conduct Disorder may also be present but that the available evidence is inconclusive. (It is worth noting that in contrast to DSM-IV-TR, DSM-5 allows for the simultaneous diagnosis of Oppositional Defiant Disorder and Conduct Disorder. See the DSM-IV-TR Note in Chapter 11.) "Rule out" can be thought of as a reminder or instruction to continue seeking the information that would allow a diagnosis to be conclusively identified or eliminated from consideration (for the present). Again, this is not language that is used within the DSM but that will be encountered in clinical reports and chart notes in community agencies.

consideration of particular cases, are useful in helping novices to gain an overall appreciation for the structure of DSM-5.

ORDERING OF DIAGNOSES

When multiple diagnoses are made, the accepted convention is that the diagnoses are listed in order of clinical importance or anticipated clinical attention. The first diagnosis listed usually also pertains to the reason for the evaluation. This is the conceptualization or understanding of the presenting problem(s) that led to the assessment. In some cases, however, the first (most significant) diagnosis will not be the reason for the evaluation. In these instances, the manual directs the examiner to note "(Principal Diagnosis)" or "(Reason for Visit)" after the diagnosis associated with the referral (see the following Application Note).

DEGREE OF DIAGNOSTIC CONFIDENCE

The manual allows for varying degrees of confidence versus uncertainty in arriving at a particular diagnosis. In an uncertain case, a diagnosis can be given, followed by the specifier "(Provisional)" to indicate less certainty in the diagnosis. For example, a diagnosis of Oppositional Defiant Disorder requires a pattern of at least four of eight symptoms of angry/irritable mood, argumentative/defiant behavior, or vindictiveness over at least 6 months. If there is clear evidence of three of the eight symptoms and an indication of a fourth symptom without clear documentation of it, the diagnosis of "Oppositional Defiant Disorder (Provisional)" may be given.

Application Note. "Principal Diagnosis"/"Reason for Visit"

In identifying which of several diagnoses given is the reason for the evaluation, there are two conventions. First, if nothing further is specified, then it is assumed that the diagnosis listed first corresponds to the reason for assessment. Second, if another diagnosis is the reason for the contact, this is noted with one of two phrases: "(Reason for Visit)" in an outpatient setting or "(Principal Diagnosis)" in a hospital or other inpatient setting. "(Principal Diagnosis)" identifies the reason for a hospital admission when a child or adolescent has several diagnoses and the decision to hospitalize the young person is not based on the diagnosis listed first. Despite this differentiation, the reader will quickly discover that the phrase "(Principal Diagnosis)" is often used by many professionals in both inpatient and outpatient settings to mark the reason for the contact.

The key point in using "(Provisional)" is that the examiner believes that the required characteristics *are* probably present and that further data will substantiate this likelihood. This designation can be contrasted with the use of Other Specified or Unspecified Disruptive Behavior Disorder. When the examiner gives a diagnosis of Other Specified or Unspecified Disruptive Behavior Disorder, he or she is convinced that there is evidence of a Mental Disorder and that the general type of Mental Disorder meets the essential features of a Disruptive Behavior Disorder; however, the examiner is not convinced that additional information will conform to the pattern of Oppositional Defiant Disorder (or another defined Disruptive Behavior Disorder).

HOW TO RECORD DIAGNOSES

Diagnostic categories in DSM-5 are defined by diagnostic criteria and identified by titles (e.g., Bulimia Nervosa). Associated with each diagnostic category are two numeric codes. The first, a four- or five- digit number—three digits followed by either one or two decimal places (e.g., 307.51)—provides the code used in the *International Classification of Diseases, 9th Revision, Clinical Modification* (ICD-9-CM) for the particular Mental Disorder. The second, a four-character alphanumeric code—a letter followed by two digits, then another after a decimal point—provides the code used in the *International Classification of Diseases, 10th Revision* (ICD-10) for that disorder. The decision to include both the ninth- and tenth-edition codes recognized that practitioners have not yet transitioned to routinely using the tenth edition, but the authors of the DSM-5 anticipated that they will soon. The ICD-9-CM and ICD-10 codes are found with diagnostic criteria (e.g., "307.51 (F50.2) Bulimia Nervosa," p. 345) or in a coding note within the diagnostic criteria when the code depends on which specifiers are present (e.g., the ICD-9-CM code for Anorexia Nervosa is 307.1; the ICD-10 code for this disorder depends on the subtype: (F50.01) for Anorexia Nervosa Restricting Type or (F50.02) Anorexia Nervosa Binge-Eating/Purging Type, p. 339). In addition, the disorder titles, ICD-9-CM codes, and ICD-10 codes for all diagnoses are given in the summary overview ("DSM-5 Classification," pp. xiii–xl) and in an Appendix providing the "Alphabetical Listing of DSM-5 Diagnoses and Codes (ICD-9-CM and ICD-10)," pp. 839–862). These codes are also listed numerically in separate appendices for each of these coding systems on pages 863–876 for the ICD-9-CM and on pages 877–896 for ICD-10.

All DSM-5 diagnoses are legitimate ICD-9-CM diagnoses, but this does not mean that all DSM-5 categories can be found in ICD-9-CM. A review of the ICD-9-CM appendix reveals that a number of DSM-5 diagnoses have the same numerical code; that is, some of the differentiations made in DSM-5 are collapsed into a single ICD-9-CM category. A similar pattern is found with the relation between DSM-5 and ICD-10 codes. There are also diagnoses available in ICD-9-CM and ICD-10 that do not appear in DSM-5. The DSM-5 Other Specified and Unspecified Disorder diagnoses for the relevant problem areas are often used to diagnose these cases. As another example, a greater selection of "V codes" (diagnostic categories that are not Mental Disorders but may be of clinical importance) is available in ICD-9-CM than in DSM-5. All submissions for insurance or government reimbursement must be made in terms of the ICD-9-CM numerical codes (soon to be transitioned to ICD-10 codes when they are implemented in the United States; see Coding Note: Implementation of ICD-10 in Chapter 3). These codes are conveniently included in DSM-5, and for most purposes it is not necessary for a school psychologist to have a copy of ICD-9-CM.

As mentioned previously, sometime soon the U.S. Department of Health and Human Services will begin requiring the use of codes from the *International Classification of Diseases, 10th Revision* (ICD-10). Several versions of ICD-10 have already been published. The ICD-10 significantly expands the number of available codes, both for Mental Disorders and for General Medical Conditions. The mechanics of this expansion of categories involve a shift from pure numerical codes (001–999) to alphanumerical codes (A00–Z99). As with ICD-9, most of the codes pertaining to mental health problems are still found in Chapter V, but the ICD-10 codes begin with the letter F (rather than falling between 290 and 319, as they do in ICD-9). Bulimia Nervosa, for instance, is coded as F50.2 in ICD-10. All DSM-5 categories are legitimate diagnoses in ICD-10, although, again, there is not perfect correspondence. ICD-10, for example, has a diagnostic category "Bulimia nervosa, atypical, F50.3" (World Health Organization, 1993) that is not found in DSM-5. (It would probably be classified as Other Specified Eating Disorder, Bulimia Nervosa [of Low Frequency and Limited Duration].)

INTERPRETATION OF DIAGNOSTIC IMPRESSIONS FROM OTHER SOURCES

Because the goal of a diagnostic classification is to communicate as much information about a child or adolescent as possible, it is valuable in making such a classification to take into consideration the information conveyed by other professionals in their diagnostic formulations. The school psychologist is often in the position of analyzing data from a variety of sources and perspectives. These data routinely include the reports of parents, teachers, and other adults working in a school setting, as well as scores on behavior rating scales, results of cognitive and academic achievement testing, scores from standardized testing in the classroom, grades, and interviews with the child. They also increasingly include reports from professionals outside the school system. Independent psychological evaluations from clinical or school psychologists; speech and audiology reports; discharge summaries or case notes from neurologists, neurosurgeons, and psychiatrists; social history reports from juvenile court officers; chemical dependence program evaluations—all of these materials may become part of the school psychologist's database for a child or adolescent. Some of these professionals will use the format of DSM-5 to communicate their summary impressions of the child's situation; others will pass along impressions from third-party sources expressed in the language of the DSM. Many school psychologists will already be familiar with the wide variability of practice in the clinical use of DSM-5 among professionals from a variety of disciplines. This access can be a motivating influence for each of us to be as clear as possible in our own diagnostic formulations and to document the data we think indicate the signs and symptoms supporting these diagnostic impressions.

At least in the short term, it is likely that, when reviewing old records, an examiner will need to deal with diagnoses from previous versions of the DSM (i.e., DSM-IV, DSM-IV-TR). The first appendix in DSM-5 provides a general discussion of changes in diagnostic categories from the fourth edition to the fifth edition of the DSM (pp. 809–816), Appendix D of DSM-IV-TR, "Annotated Listing of Changes in DSM-IV" (pp. 829–843 there), served the same purpose. We continue to find it valuable on occasion to have copies of earlier editions of the DSM available in our offices.

Part II

GUIDELINES FOR EVALUATION OF PRESENTING PROBLEMS

INTRODUCTION

Evaluation of a child or adolescent referred for psychological services begins with the presenting problems that have brought the young person to professional attention. Most often, the youth's adult caretakers have voiced some concerns regarding his or her actions, performance, and/or emotions. Thus begins the process of diagnostic formulation. Presenting concerns both raise diagnostic possibilities and suggest areas of investigation to refine diagnostic hypotheses. As further data are gathered, the clinical picture of the young person's adjustment is developed in greater and greater detail. The goal of diagnostic classification is to recognize the most important patterns within the assessment data and to assign the diagnosis or diagnoses that best capture the most helpful information about the child's or adolescent's adjustment, functioning, and problems.

In this part of the book, some of the most common presenting concerns of caretakers are reviewed with respect to how DSM-5 diagnoses can be assigned to these problems. The organization of this discussion is thematic. Beginning with a broad area of concern—that is, acting out or externalizing behavior problems—the diagnostic categories of potential relevance are discussed. Initial consideration is usually given to the most salient categories or the ones most frequently applied; alternative possibilities with lower base rates are then discussed in turn. Usually, possible diagnoses drawn from multiple chapters within DSM-5 are reviewed, because a human problem is seldom so simple and straightforward that one and only one diagnostic formulation will be apparent from the first contact. A common source of confusion and frustration among our first-year graduate students as they begin to learn the DSM-5 system is that "You have to know it all just to begin." Indeed, the examiner does need a general familiarity with the total classification system and with the logic of the system, because differential diagnoses from several areas within DSM-5 may need to be considered for each case. DSM-5 itself tries to address this difficulty with the "Differential Diagnosis" section for each diagnosis. First (2014) draws together material on differential diagnostic considerations to assist the evaluator in thinking about the most likely choices and to highlight the critical points of differences among diagnoses under consideration. We hope that the organization of this book helps the reader develop a rapid familiarity with the DSM-5 framework and that this understanding will assist in the efficient use of the classification system.

To help accomplish this goal, it has been necessary to keep the text relatively brief. This brevity has been accomplished in several ways. Some of the discussions of specific diagnoses are quite short, even when a great deal is known about the pattern, course, and variant expressions of a problem. In fact, especially when a great deal is known about a problem and the problem is generally well understood by most practicing psychologists, this common knowledge is not reiterated. The purpose here is not to give a general discussion of behavioral and emotional problems in youth. There are several good texts on child psychopathology; in particular, Mash and Barkley (2014) use DSM as the framework for discussing the assessment and treatment of childhood problems. In this part of this volume, we describe the categories of DSM-5, attempt to clarify the diagnostic issues involved, and show how clinical information can be represented within DSM-5.

Another departure from many professional presentations is that referencing is intentionally sparse. Relatively noncontroversial statements regarding behavior problems are simply presented. The references that are given have usually been selected because they provide particularly pertinent results, because they represent recent empirical research, or occasionally because of their classic status within the history of psychology. Opinions and conclusions based on our own personal professional experiences are identified as such to the best of our abilities.

5

Problems with Intellectual Ability and Cognition

OVERVIEW

Problems with intellectual ability and cognition receive primary focus in DSM-5 in three areas: Intellectual Disability (Intellectual Developmental Disorder; formerly Mental Retardation), Global Developmental Delay, and Neurocognitive Disorders. (A V code, Borderline Intellectual Functioning, may also be applicable in some cases.) The first two areas are found in the Neurodevelopmental Disorders chapter of DSM-5, whereas the third is covered in a separate chapter on Neurocognitive Disorders, which includes coverage of what were previously known as Organic Mental Disorders. The applied psychologist is well prepared to contribute to the assessment of children in these areas, although the use of the diagnoses for neurocognitive problems in DSM-5 (e.g., Delirium) may be one of the greatest "stretches" for the practicing school psychologist.

It is worth recognizing that intellectual functioning is one of the few areas in DSM-5 in which formal psychological assessment is mentioned or prescribed. Yet even here, the emphasis remains on the clinical assessment and judgment of the examiner. Formal testing may set limits within which judgment takes place, but it does not replace or supplant the primary responsibility of the examiner in determining the most appropriate diagnostic classification. Independent of its other strengths or weaknesses, DSM-5, like its predecessors, is about assessment and not testing.

INTELLECTUAL DISABILITY AND RELATED PROBLEMS

Definitions and Subclassification of Intellectual Disability

Intellectual Disability, formerly known as Mental Retardation (see the Author Commentary below), requires little discussion with regard to making a DSM-5 diagnosis. The school psychologist will find that the conceptualization of Intellectual Disability in DSM-5 is quite familiar because it is based on the original tripartite conception of the former American Association on Mental Deficiency (Grossman, 1983; Heber, 1959, 1961): subnormal intellectual functioning, impairment in adaptive behavior in one or more domains, and onset during childhood or adolescence. (See the next Application Note: Intellectual Disability and Development: Age-of-Onset Criterion.) Unlike most other diagnostic categories in DSM-5, standardized testing is explicitly required for diagnosis of Intellectual Disability. In this case, DSM-5 requires individual, standardized testing that generates an IQ that is at least 2 standard deviations below the mean (±5 points for error in measurement). This criterion is consistent with other systems of classification in terms of the intellectual deficits.

Author Commentary. Labeling Intellectual Disability

We both think the name change from "Mental Retardation" to "Intellectual Disability" was unfortunate and ill advised (we had much more colorful adjectives, but the editor and lawyers made us take them out). The authors of DSM-5 say the change reflects the fact that the term "mental retardation" has become pejorative and hurtful. They are absolutely right in this observation. Their solution was to use a new "name" that is clinically neutral and will not cause hurt feelings. If you had no understanding at all of the history of mental health, you might think this name change would work. It will not. We make this statement with such finality because it has been tried before, repeatedly, and it has never worked. There was a time when "idiot," "imbecile," and "moron" were clinical terms used to discuss degrees of cognitive disadvantage; these terms quickly became the verbal rocks thrown at in-laws and politicians. These hurtful and pejorative terms were replaced with neutral clinical descriptions, such as "mentally defective," which in turn became hurtful and were replaced with "mental retardation." An early attempt to sanitize the language advocated replacing "mental retardation" with "developmental disability." Shortly after this name replacement began, one of us heard a child call another on the playground: "You DD."

The problem is not the term. "Mental retardation" is a perfectly acceptable and accurate description of the phenomenon under discussion. The common characteristic of the vast majority of individuals with intellectual disabilities is not what they learn or are capable of doing, but how rapidly they can learn and under what circumstances they will acquire a skill. Their learning is slower, and they benefit more than most from optimal teaching approaches. We argue that this term is, on the face of it, much more descriptive and less inherently limiting than "intellectual disability."

The real problem is that we need to face up to the reality of individual differences—we are not all alike. This reality brings both interest and possibilities to the world and also the opportunities for prejudice, discrimination, stereotyping, and other problems. We struggle with differences that make little actual difference, such as skin tone. It is perhaps not surprising that we have problems with differences that actually have real-world implications, such as cognitive ability. Until we come to terms with what we want to make of differences in conceptual facility, whatever term we use for the low end of the distribution will quickly be absorbed by our culture as another "verbal rock" to throw at people who upset us. The change of terminology from "Mental Retardation" to "Intellectual Disability" is a cosmetic solution to a deeper issue. The cost is that this change allows us to pretend we have fixed a problem when we really have not done anything of substance at all. With that being said, the terminology has changed, and practitioners will need to move to the new wording.

Application Note. Intellectual Disability and Development: Age-of-Onset Criterion

Unlike previous editions of DSM, the fifth edition has dropped the criterion of age of onset before 18 years in favor of the more common criterion of onset during the developmental period. For the practicing school psychologist, this change more closely aligns the DSM definition of Intellectual Disability with that detailed in IDEA, as well as the definition adopted by AAIDD. The DSM further allows the diagnosis of Intellectual Disability to be assigned along with other acquired forms of deficits (e.g., traumatic brain injury or other neurocognitive disorder) if both are present during the developmental period. It also recognizes that early and ongoing intervention and supports can lead to the removal of the diagnosis.

The subclassification of Intellectual Disability in DSM-5 is based solely on the severity of adaptive functioning deficits (see the following Application Note). In response to the most recently revised definition of Intellectual Disability by the American Association on Intellectual and Developmental Disabilities (AAIDD; Schalock et al., 2010), DSM-5 has based decisions about subclassification on level of adaptive functioning deficits, not cognitive ability. That is, users are to specify severity based on functioning in conceptual, social, and practical domains (see the following Professional Note). It is important to note that DSM-5 does not provide guidance for decision rules when functioning in one or more domains is different from that in others. It merely encourages examiners to use clinical judgment in these determinations (see the next Author Commentary on page 43).

Application Note. DSM-5 Subclassification of Intellectual Disability: Degrees of Severity

The DSM-5 subclassification of Intellectual Disability is based on level of functioning in the conceptual, social, and practical domains. It identifies four specific groups largely defined by the level of supports required: Mild, Moderate, Severe, and Profound. DSM-5 also provides some guidance in terms of presentation at different stages of development. Preschoolers classified as mild in severity may demonstrate little or no differences in the conceptual domain, but as they progress in school, difficulty in learning will likely become apparent. In adulthood, deficits in applying academic skills are likely to be seen, along with relatively concrete rather than abstract thinking. Within the social domain, individuals classified as Mild in severity will likely appear immature and less skilled in their communication, language, conversation, and emotion regulation relative to their peers. For individuals classified with the Mild severity specifier, differences in the practical domain will likely be less apparent until adulthood, when supports are often needed for medical, legal, vocational, and child-rearing responsibilities.

Classification at the Moderate severity level is specified for preschoolers who demonstrate delayed language and preacademic skills. As they move forward in school, children classified in the Moderate range show slow progress in the major academic areas (i.e., reading, writing, mathematics) and in comprehending money and time. For individuals at the Moderate severity level, conceptual development is expected to peak at the elementary-school level. Thus, support is needed for daily conceptual tasks. Within the social domain, marked differences are expected in communication and social skills relative to typical peers. These differences are likely to be apparent in all relationships and to require support to maintain employment and to make life decisions. Within the practical domain, prolonged training and support is usually needed to allow the individual to achieve independence in personal needs (e.g., hygiene, toileting, eating, dressing). In adulthood, employment is possible with additional supports from supervisors, coworkers, and others. Maladaptive behavior may be present in a minority of individuals who are assigned the Moderate specifier.

The Severe specifier is assigned to individuals with limited conceptual and communication skills who have little understanding of written language, time, and money. Individuals classified with the Severe specifier require extensive supports throughout the lifespan, including assistance with all activities of daily living (e.g., hygiene, eating, eliminating) and decision making. Maladaptive behavior is present in a sizable minority of individuals who are assigned the Severe specifier.

The Profound specifier is assigned to individuals who have conceptual skills limited to concrete objects. Communication for individuals with this specifier is largely nonverbal and nonsymbolic. In terms of practical support needs, the Profound specifier indicates extensive assistance required in all aspects of daily life. Co-occurring physical and sensory impairments, as well as maladaptive behavior, are observed in this subcategory.

Beyond this main diagnosis, there are three closely related DSM-5 categories: Global Developmental Delay, Unspecified Intellectual Disability, and Borderline Intellectual Functioning. Diagnosis of Global Developmental Delay is restricted to children at or below 5 years old whose clinical severity cannot be reliably assessed. In contrast, diagnosis of Unspecified Intellectual Disability is appropriate only for individuals over the age of 5 years whose abilities are difficult or impossible to assess because of sensory, motor, behavioral, and/or mental health issues. Thus, Unspecified Intellectual Disability is used to cover cases in which there is strong presumptive evidence of Intellectual Disability but in which an acceptable measure of intellectual functioning is not available (the client cannot be tested, is uncooperative, or is otherwise impossible to assess). The availability of this diagnosis both gives DSM-5 considerable flexibility and challenges the intellectual honesty of the examiner, although its intent is not to give an "easy out" in cases that present an assessment challenge. It is left to the examiner to determine when a given child or adolescent (or adult) cannot be validly assessed with quantitative instruments that have acceptable psychometric qualities.

In keeping with DSM-5's attempt to adopt a dimensional, empirical approach to diagnosis, it also includes a V-code for Borderline Intellectual Functioning. This category is appropriate for individuals for whom cognitive and adaptive functioning are relevant to treatment but for whom the criteria for Intellectual Disability are not met.

Author Commentary. Levels of Severity for Intellectual Disability

Typically, past systems of classification of Intellectual Disability have been subclassified on the basis of severity. This practice continues in DSM-5, but the assessment of severity has changed. Whereas past classifications in the DSM were based on tested IQ, the current approach is to classify into Mild, Moderate, Severe, and Profound on the basis of considering three areas of adaptive functioning: Conceptual, Social, and Practical. Table 1 on pages 34–36 in DSM-5 provides a matrix of descriptions of each of these areas of adaptive functioning for each level of severity. The rationale for this change is that it is adaptive functioning rather than tested intelligence that determines the level of support needed. This critical status of adaptive behavior was also the rationale for the movement away from IQ levels in recent editions of the AAIDD classifications (Schalock et al., 2010). The DSM text also asserts that IQ measures are less valid in the lower range of scores. This second assertion is debatable—we would argue that intellectual deficits are in fact more stable and valid in the lowest range but that our measures of these low scores are poor. Perhaps this distinction is quibbling. Be that as it may, DSM has gone with clinical judgments of adaptive behavior (over any number of alternative measures: Inventory for Client and Agency Planning, Vineland Adaptive Behavior Scales, Scales of Independent Behavior, Adaptive Behavior Assessment System), which is fine, and they give us a matrix to help consider the three areas they focus on, which is also fine, *but they don't tell us how to use it.*

Suppose there are disagreements in our judgment of the child's performance in the three areas: Profound on Conceptual, Mild on Social, Moderate on Practical. What should we do? How do we assign the degree of severity? Any number of perfectly reasonable decision rules could have been offered: (1) Take the highest; an aspirational argument and some data could be offered here. (2) Take the lowest; we need to know the most limiting factors. (3) Take an average, either informally or by assigning values to the level and doing a rough calculation. (4) Assign priority to one of the three areas or give a rank ordering of priority (e.g., practicality is most significant in long-term outcome, so use this rating in case of disagreements; we recognize that different arguments could be advanced for each of the three areas). Any of these would have "worked" in terms of giving clear guidance about how to adjudicate among disagreements. We all might have had a favorite answer and been happy or sad depending on whether this preference had been picked, but regardless of the outcome we would have known how we were supposed to be making this determination. Instead, we are left to make a clinical determination. The authors of the DSM emphasize the need for clinical decision making and clinical responsibility. We fully agree with this assertion, but this determination was not the place to rely on that. It was the place to make a decision. Tell us all how it is to be done, and observe how it works out in preparation for DSM 5.1 or 6 or whatever. We predict that the absence of a clear decision rule here will contribute to impressionistic (and unreliable) judgments.

Professional Note. Intellectual Disability as Defined by DSM-5 and the AAIDD

Both the AAIDD and the DSM-5 definitions of Intellectual Disability retain the three basic elements articulated in the previous original formulation: significant subaverage intellectual functioning, related limitations in adaptive skill areas, and onset during the developmental period. Relative to previous editions of the DSM, however, the DSM-5 definition of Intellectual Disability is better aligned with the AAIDD conception of Intellectual Disability. That is, DSM-5, like AAIDD, gives priority to deficits in adaptive functioning in one or more activities of daily living as opposed to intellectual functioning when determining eligibility. Thus, an even greater emphasis is placed on deficits in adaptive behavior, and subclassification is based on the intensity of supports needed to maintain maximum adaptation in individuals with Intellectual Disability.

The practical implications of these seemingly subtle shifts of emphasis are potentially quite significant. Greater attention to adaptive behavior creates an even greater need for valid and reliable measures of this important domain of adjustment. The possibility that an individual with a tested IQ of between 70 and 75 (and clinically significant impairment in adaptive behavior) might be classified as having Intellectual Disability could potentially affect the official classification of a vast population of citizens. Basing the subclassification of Intellectual Disability on level of support rather than tested intelligence not only is a fundamental shift away from the standard practice used with previous classification systems but also demands a methodology that has not yet been established as reliable or valid. As with previous editions of the DSM, the four degrees of Intellectual Disability severity are given fuzzy boundaries. No guidance is provided in terms of how to weight the three domains of functioning to determine diagnosis and subclassification. Diagnosis requires deficits or impaired effectiveness in at least one activity of daily living, but determination of these deficits is left up to the judgment of the examiner. The school psychologist should note that DSM-5 now matches other diagnostic systems in terms of the age-of-origin criterion, namely, within the developmental period.

IDEA Note. Intellectual Disability and IDEA

Intellectual Disability is an identified qualifying condition for special education services under IDEA. This apparently straightforward statement is complicated, however, by variation in the meaning of "intellectual disability" across the various documents and practices. The children identified by various state definitions as showing subaverage general intelligence may or may not qualify for a DSM-5 diagnosis of Intellectual Disability, which is a Mental Disorder. Children showing tested subaverage intellectual and adaptive functioning that is relevant to treatment are assigned the DSM-5 V code of Borderline Intellectual Functioning, which is not a Mental Disorder category. Some of these children, especially these at the lower end of the range, will probably qualify for special education services under the IDEA classification of "intellectual disability." The situation is further confused by the apparent tendency of some school districts to classify some children who show the general pattern of Mild Intellectual Disability under the alternative conceptualization of "learning disabled" (Gresham, MacMillan, & Bocian, 1998; Gresham, MacMillan, & Siperstein, 1995).

It is worth considering that advances in understanding the genetic, physiological, and neurological bases of Intellectual Disability may finally result in improved clarity in our views of this large and highly heterogeneous population (see State, King, & Dykens, 1997). In their review, King, State, Shah, Davanzo, and Dykens (1997, p. 1662) note that Intellectual Disability "ranks first among chronic conditions that cause major limitations in activity for persons in the United States (Centers for Disease Control [and Prevention], 1996)." Staying abreast of these developments will be one of the exciting challenges for school and clinical psychologists in the 21st century. The previous IDEA Note sets forth how Intellectual Disability relates to eligibility for services under IDEA, and the following Professional Note discusses how Intellectual Disability relates to expectations for educability.

Professional Note. Intellectual Disability and Educability Expectations

The only serious competition to the traditional five-category model of "intellectual disability" in psychiatry (borderline, mild, moderate, severe, profound) was the three-category model (educable, trainable, custodial), which was defined by measured cognitive ability. It evolved in education to help set educability expectations for what were then termed "mentally handicapped children." The original purpose of this diagnostic system was to establish responsibility for care. Prior to the passage of Public Law 94-142, many children classified as trainable and probably all classified as custodial were excluded from a free public education. Public Law 94-142 (and IDEA, which supplanted it) redefined the term "education" from a narrow focus on academic skills to a broader conception that included the development of adaptive behavior. This change led to the inclusion of most children with intellectual disability within public education, and the functional significance of the educational classification system was greatly reduced. One version of this system is discussed in Hardman, Drew, and Egan (2014). They identify the Educable range as having a tested IQ of 55 to about 70 and the Trainable range as a tested IQ of 40 to about 55.

Borderline Intellectual Functioning

It is worth reiterating that Borderline Intellectual Functioning is not a Mental Disorder in the language of DSM-5. Instead, it is one of the categories in the chapter titled "Other Conditions That May Be a Focus of Clinical Attention" (see the Coding Note)—behavior problems and other complications that may justify clinical evaluation and treatment but that do not fall within the definition of Mental Disorders in DSM-5. The title of the chapter in which it appears suggests that the limited cognitive and adaptive abilities have some deleterious consequences in the individual's life. The school psychologist will find that the V codes in general are both indispensably useful in assessing children and adolescents and extremely frustrating in their lack of specificity and objectivity. Unfortunately, there are no criterion sets for the V codes to help encourage their consistent application.

Associated Problems and Diagnoses

Children with low intellectual functioning are at elevated risk for other behavior problems (Einfeld, Ellis, & Emerson, 2011; Harris, 2006; Whitaker & Read, 2006; Yoo, Valdovinos, & Schroeder, 2012). Greater than base-rate prevalences for aggressive behavior, self-injurious behaviors, stereotypic behaviors, overactivity, and language problems are reported for children and adolescents diagnosed with Intellectual Disability (Aman,

Coding Note. "V Codes"

In DSM-III and DSM-III-R, the codes for all of the categories in the "Other Conditions That May Be a Focus of Clinical Attention" section began with the letter V. This practice was no longer completely the case with DSM-IV or with DSM-5, but the informal designation continues to be commonly used. A V code is a diagnosis, but it is not a diagnosis of a Mental Disorder. It is a diagnosis of a condition that justifies professional response but that does not meet the defining criteria for a Mental Disorder.

Hammer, & Rojahn, 1993; Bregman, 1991; Jacobson, 1982; Scott, 1994). A 6-year study of individuals with what is now diagnosed as Intellectual Disability found "the entire range of psychiatric diagnoses" represented (Menolascino, 1988, p. 111), including a significant overrepresentation of Schizophrenia (DSM-III criteria). Instead of explaining these problems away as part of the disability, educators will serve young people with Intellectual Disability better by recognizing their associated mental health problems and treating these emotional and behavioral disturbances whenever possible. An examiner must realize that there is nothing about Intellectual Disability that protects a young person from other behavior problems, even if these are not differentially associated with Intellectual Disability. A negative change in a child's or adolescent's level of adjustment should lead to a high index of suspicion in the examiner regarding possible new difficulties, either environmental stresses or comorbid mental disorders. In our experiences with clients with developmental disabilities, we have seen both Major Depressive Episodes and Manic Episodes that were missed in evaluations, despite obvious deteriorations in performance. The clients' significant problems with depression and agitation were not recognized as potential indications of treatable disorders—sometimes with disastrous results.

In Mild to Moderate Intellectual Disability, the other diagnostic categories of DSM-5 have reasonable applicability, although even this statement is not as well supported with empirical data as would be desirable. With increasing severity of intellectual deficit, however, there is concern regarding the validity of categories developed primarily for individuals with intelligence in the average range (Einfeld & Aman, 1995). At the same time, the likelihood of associated behavior and emotional problems appears to increase with increasing severity of Intellectual Disability (Campbell & Malone, 1991; Einfeld & Aman, 1995; Einfeld et al., 2011). In our work with children and adolescents with Intellectual Disability, we have often had occasion to use residual (Unspecified Intellectual Disability) diagnoses. Einfeld and Aman (1995) suggest that multivariate analyses of behavioral and emotional symptoms in youth with Intellectual Disability yield some consistent dimensions of disturbance. Potentially relevant diagnoses from DSM-5 pertaining to these areas are shown in Table 5.1.

Several authors have discussed modifications of the DSM diagnostic criteria to increase their sensitivity and applicability to comorbid mental disorders in individuals with Intellectual Disability (King, DeAntonio, McCracken, Forness, & Ackerland, 1994; Reiss, 1994; Szymanski, 1994). As with any modification of the DSM-5 diagnostic criteria, the examiner has the responsibility of being clear and explicit about the basis on which a diagnosis is being made. Kay (1989) suggested that psychometric testing could be useful in making a differential diagnosis between Intellectual Disability and psychosis, but we are not aware of replication of this work.

King and colleagues (1994) comment that many individuals with a diagnosis of Intellectual Disability do not fit neatly into a single diagnostic category. Comorbidity among different diagnoses is quite common, as are subsyndromal presentations. A young person with Intellectual Disability may show features of a Mood or Anxiety Disorder that do not meet full criteria for a diagnosis but do substantially interfere with his or her adjustment and complicate the case. Provisional and "rule-out" diagnoses are often found in the charts of clients with Intellectual Disability (King et al., 1994). As we have noted before, the use of the Unspecified classification within the major DSM-5 diagnostic groupings has proved helpful in our work with children and adolescents with Intellectual Disability who show other behavioral problems.

A few disorders that commonly co-occur with Intellectual Disability are worth mentioning specifically. Stereotypic movements (motor behaviors that are repetitive, nonfunctional, and self-stimulatory) are often seen in association with Intellectual Disability, especially as the severity of Intellectual Disability increases (Campbell & Malone, 1991); if such behaviors become troublesome enough to justify a treatment focus, the diagnosis of Stereotypic Movement Disorder (discussed in Chapter 6) can be made concurrently with that of Intellectual Disability. The specifier With Self-Injurious Behavior is noted if applicable and would also accompany the Associated with a Known Neurodevelopmental Disorder specifier. Self-injurious behavior is associated both with the severity of Intellectual Disability and with environmental influences (Campbell & Malone, 1991).

A diagnosis of Intellectual Disability can be made concurrently with a diagnosis of Autism Spectrum Disorder, and in fact these are commonly comorbid conditions (see Chapter 7). DSM-5 notes that Autism Spectrum Disorder is frequently associated with impaired intellectual functioning (p. 40). A child who shows Intellectual Disability, Autism Spectrum Disorder, and repetitive self-injurious behavior should not receive an additional diagnosis of Stereotypic Movement Disorder, unless it involves self-injurious behavior that has become a significant focus of clinical attention.

TABLE 5.1. DSM-5 Diagnoses to Be Considered in Regard to Other Symptoms of Disturbance in Populations with Intellectual Disability

Area of disturbance	Diagnoses/conditions to be ruled in/out
Neurodevelopmental	Attention-Deficit/Hyperactivity Disorder (ADHD) Other Specified or Unspecified ADHD
Aggressive or antisocial behavior	Oppositional Defiant Disorder Intermittent Explosive Disorder Conduct Disorder Other Specified Disruptive, Impulse-Control, and Conduct Disorder Unspecified Disruptive, Impulse-Control, and Conduct Disorder Adjustment Disorder with Disturbance of Conduct Adjustment Disorder with Mixed Disturbance of Emotions and Conduct Child or Adolescent Antisocial Behavior—the possibility the behavior is not a Mental Disorder
Social withdrawal	Autism Spectrum Disorder Social Anxiety Disorder (Social Phobia) Unspecified Anxiety Disorder Adjustment Disorder with Anxiety Adjustment Disorder with Anxiety and Depressed Mood
Mood	Disruptive Mood Regulation Disorder Major Depressive Disorder Persistent Depressive Disorder Premenstrual Dysphoric Disorder Unspecified Depressive Disorder Adjustment Disorder with Depressed Mood Bipolar Disorder Cyclothymic Disorder
Obsessive–Compulsive and Related Disorders	Obsessive–Compulsive Disorder Hoarding Disorder Trichotillomania (Hair-Pulling Disorder) Excoriation (Skin-Picking) Disorder
Feeding and Eating Disorders	Pica Rumination Disorder
Elimination Disorders	Enuresis Encopresis
Motor Disorders	Stereotypic Movement Disorder Tourette's Disorder Persistent (Chronic) Motor or Vocal Tic Disorder
Unspecified Personality Disorder	
Unspecified Mental Disorder (nonpsychotic)	

In some cases, a person diagnosed with Intellectual Disability may experience a later decline in his or her level of mental ability. These new challenges would be diagnosed as a neurocognitive disorder in addition to the preexisting Intellectual Disability. Considering pragmatic issues in determining premorbid level of functioning, DSM-5 suggests that a concurrent diagnosis of Major Neurocognitive Disorder (formerly Dementia in DSM-IV-TR) with Intellectual Disability only be used for those cases in which the essential features of the clinical situation are not adequately captured by the solitary diagnosis of Intellectual Disability. For example, an individual with Trisomy 21, a genetic condition asssociated with Intellectual Disability, will develop Alzheimer's Disease in middle adulthood and experience additional loss of mental capability. This decline would appropriately be diagnosed as a Major Neurocognitive Disorder (Dementia) and Intellectual Disability.

NEUROCOGNITIVE DISORDERS

The Neurocognitive Disorders chapter of DSM-5 covers clinically significant deficits in mental ability that represent a change from a previous level of functioning. These disorders were referred to as Organic Mental Disorders in DSM-III-R; this label was dropped because of concern that it implied an absence of biological basis for "nonorganic" mental disorders. Strub and Black (1988) suggested the designation of "neurobehavioral disorders" for these biologically based problems of mental processing, but the authors of DSM-IV opted out of advancing a summary label in favor of a chapter titled, "Delirium, Dementia, and Amnestic and Other Cognitive Disorders." In DSM-5, the authors selected a title similar to that suggested by Strub and Black. This chapter, in contrast with other DSM-5 chapters, captures pathology for which there are potentially known causes that occur later in development. These categories have their most common applications with adults, but because several possible applications pertain to children and adolescents, the school psychologist should have some knowledge of this group of diagnoses.

Delirium

Delirium involves acute disturbances in consciousness and cognition. Strub and Black (1988) label these disorders "acute confusional states," which conveys a clear picture of the problem, but the more traditional term remains popular and is used in DSM-5. Delirium in children and adolescents presents in the context of serious medical conditions that bring the youth into a health care setting.

Major and Mild Neurocognitive Disorder

What was previously referred to as "Dementia" is relabeled in DSM-5 as a Major Neurocognitive Disorder. This disorder involves a loss of previously established mental ability. In DSM-5, a Major Neurocognitive Disorder is defined by a demonstrable decline from previous performances in one or more areas of cognitive functioning: complex attention, executive functioning, learning and memory, language, perceptual–motor, or social cognition. This definition is a significant change from the DSM-IV standard of a decline in memory plus one other affected area of cognitive ability and is consistent with the overall literature on dementias: Memory is often, but not always, the first area of impairment. The Neurocognitive Disorders categories identify a pattern of cognitive deficits without assumption about the course or stability of these impairments. DSM-5 then further differentiates the Major and Mild Neurocognitive Disorders by presumed etiology. This distinction may often overstep our current diagnostic ability, but it continues the precedence of DSM-IV.

Of special interest to the school psychologist is Major or Mild Neurocognitive Disorder Due to Traumatic Brain Injury, an unacceptably frequent occurrence in school-age individuals. Major or Mild Neurocognitive Disorder Due to Another Medical Condition (e.g., lead encephalopathy) are also seen in school settings. In addition, it may be useful for the school psychologist to be aware of associations between Neurocognitive Disorders and other medical disorders of relevance to educators. For instance, it appears that all individuals with trisomy 21 (Down syndrome), a common etiology of Intellectual Disability, will develop the neurological characteristics of Alzheimer's disease in their adult lives (Pietrini et al., 1997).

The insistence on associating Major and Mild Neurocognitive Disorders with specific etiologies is consistent with the increased biological emphasis in DSM-5, but examiners will frequently be unable to clearly establish the causes of disorders, especially in early stages of evaluation. Definitive diagnoses of etiology often require invasive evaluations, such as samples of brain tissues, which are usually not available. Most neurocognitive diagnoses will be qualified by "probable" or "possible" and many will remain "Unspecified" or "Due to Multiple Etiologies." In contrast to establishing definite etiology, most presumptive diagnoses of neurocognitive disorders are based on symptom patterns and symptom progress and course. With sufficient effort to contact collaterals, these patterns can often be established with relative confidence. Psychological professionals usually have great expertise in this area and can make valuable contributions. Psychological and neuropsychological testing can provide useful documentation of several of the areas of cognitive functioning needed to determine Major and Mild Neurocognitive Disorders (e.g., memory, global

Etiologies →

intellectual functioning, language, perceptual–motor ability). Measures of executive functioning and social cognition are less well established but continue to be a focus of effort and development.

Mild Neurocognitive Disorders follow a similar pattern to Major Neurocognitive Disorders, but they have a lower threshold of severity (and diagnostic confidence) and do not imply compromise in independent functioning. This differentiation will often be difficult to make in adolescents and especially children, in whom full independence in adaptive behaviors of daily living is still being developed. The use of adaptive behavior scales based on retrospective and current ratings of behavior may be especially useful in this area. For most psychological examiners, the most commonly encountered Neurocognitive Disorders in youth will probably be those conditions secondary to head trauma. There is an ever-growing literature on traumatic brain injury assessment and treatment in youth (Davies, 2014). The category of Mild Neurocognitive Disorder will provide a possible formal diagnostic recognition of a "postconcussional disorder." The concept of an identifiable pattern of mental difficulty and neurobehavioral symptoms following so-called "mild head injury" (i.e., head injury without definitive neurological signs) has been investigated and discussed for several decades in the neurological and neuropsychological literature.

Unspecified Neurocognitive Disorder

Unspecified Neurocognitive Disorder is the residual classification for acquired deficits in cognitive ability that do not meet the essential features for the three identified patterns of Major and Mild Neurocognitive Disorder or Delirium. In cases of postconcussional phenomena that do not meet the diagnostic criteria for Mild Neurocognitive Disorder, this residual category is appropriate, assuming that the examiner recognizes the presentation as meeting the definition of a Mental Disorder.

Major or Mild Neurocognitive Disorder Due to Traumatic Brain Injury

The topic of traumatic brain injury has received increasing interest within school settings since the acceptance of Traumatic Brain Injury as a qualifying condition for special education services in 1990. The next IDEA Note sets forth how Traumatic Brain Injury relates to eligibility for services under IDEA. According to the Centers for Disease Control and Prevention (Faul, Xu, Wald, & Coronado, 2010), nearly half a million emergency department visits are made for traumatic brain injuries in U.S. children between 0 and 14 years old. Each year approximately 35,000 youth between the ages of 0 and 14 acquire some degree of residual disability secondary to a traumatic brain injury.

IDEA Note. Traumatic Brain Injury and IDEA

When Public Law 94-142 (Education of All Handicapped Children Act) was revised as IDEA (Public Law 101-476) in 1990, the category of traumatic brain injury was added as an identified qualifying condition establishing eligibility for special education and other services through the school system. Traumatic brain injury is not a Mental Disorder in the DSM-5 classification system, although it may be an etiological factor in several different disorders. Traumatic brain injury is a significant medical condition, and it could be an etiological factor in a Major or Mild Neurocognitive Disorder and/or most of the other Mental Disorders. Deterioration or loss in a child's or adolescent's mental functioning and/or behavioral adjustment caused by a traumatic brain injury is a Mental Disorder. Almost all children who survive the initial trauma leading to a traumatic brain injury will eventually return to school (Carney & Schoenbrodt, 1994). Their adjustment thereafter may be dramatically altered by the cognitive and emotional/behavioral consequences of the brain injury.

Traumatic brain injury in children is a risk factor for cognitive and behavioral problems (Begali, 1992; Rutter, 1981). Although the association between severe traumatic brain injury and behavioral and adaptive problems is well established (Brown, Chadwick, Shaffer, Rutter, & Traub, 1981; Fay et al., 1994; Fletcher, Ewing-Cobbs, Miner, Levin, & Eisenberg, 1990; Knights et al., 1991; Max, Smith, et al., 1997; Rivara et al., 1993), the relation between mild traumatic brain injury and psychiatric outcome has been more widely debated (Max & Dunisch, 1997). Development of a "novel" psychiatric disorder (i.e., a disorder unobserved prior to injury) during the first 3 months following a traumatic brain injury in children and adolescents is associated with greater severity of the injury, lower preinjury intellectual ability, a premorbid history of behavior problems, and a family history of psychiatric problems (Max, Smith, et al., 1997). Common initial cognitive difficulties following a traumatic brain injury include problems with general intellectual functioning, cognitive flexibility, memory, and verbal fluency (Slater & Bassett, 1988), which can have serious implications for a child's or adolescent's return to school and community. Careful assessment and follow-up by the school psychologist can greatly facilitate such a young person's successful reentry into his or her academic and social worlds. Awareness and communication of common associated symptoms of traumatic brain injury can help minimize adjustment problems. Greater vulnerability to fatigue, illness, chemical influences (prescription, over-the-counter, and illicit substances), and stress are typical sequelae of traumatic brain injury; all can have significant educational implications. The longitudinal studies of Max, Robin, and colleagues (1997) found that injury severity, preinjury family functioning, and preinjury adjustment history were all related to the continued presence of "novel" psychiatric problems during the second year following traumatic brain injury.

Although it is desirable for the school psychologist to be sensitive to the multiple potential consequences of traumatic brain injury in children, it is also necessary to recognize that a history of recent traumatic brain injury does not automatically mean that neurological insult is the causal agent in any adjustment problems. There is no unique pattern of maladjustment associated with traumatic brain injury in children; the problems seen are essentially the same as those of a general group of children with mental health difficulties (Max, Sharma, & Qurashi, 1997). Chronic problems that predate the head injury are obviously not caused by traumatic brain injury. Making the most appropriate interpretation of exacerbations of long-standing adjustment difficulties following traumatic brain injury is challenging and should usually be done cautiously. Particular caution is prudent in cases that are in or may be headed to litigation. For psychologists the important factors of a case are usually the child's current behavior and abilities and deficits and how these areas be best addressed; questions of cause or etiology are often secondary. In forensic arenas, the issue of causality is usually of pivotal concern. A hard reality is that we usually cannot be absolutely certain that two events, even when one follows the other, are causally related. We know that the child was in an accident and sustained a head injury. We know that the child is now scoring poorly on any number of cognitive or academic measures or is doing poorly in school. Whether we know "with a reasonable degree of psychological certainty" (the qualifying phrase in much forensic testimony) that the head injury caused the poor intellectual performance now seen is a different matter. We recommend caution in offering opinions on these issues, given the limits of confidence regarding causality.

6

Learning, Communication, and Motor Problems

OVERVIEW

Learning, communication, and motor problems are covered in three main areas within the Neurodevelopmental Disorders section of DSM-5: Specific Learning Disorder, Communication Disorders, and Motor Disorders. (An additional V code, Educational Problems, may also be applicable in some cases.) Applied psychologists, particularly school-based practitioners, are well versed in assessment of learning and communication difficulties, although many may find the diagnoses available for learning and communication problems within DSM-5 less than satisfying. In contrast, applied psychologists have less experience in assessing motor difficulties and may benefit from consultation with experts in an allied profession, such as physical or occupational therapists.

It is noteworthy that the assessment of learning and communication (in addition to the assessment of intellectual functioning) is the only area in DSM-5 in which formal psychological or language assessment is mentioned or prescribed. As noted in the previous chapter, the emphasis still remains on the clinical assessment and judgment of the examiner over formal testing of these areas. Formal testing provides valuable data, but it does not replace the primary responsibility of the examiner in determining the most appropriate diagnostic classification. It is a good reminder that the diagnostic process is not the rote activity of a technician but a sophisticated interplay and integration of findings used to make sense of human experience.

LEARNING DISORDERS AND RELATED PROBLEMS

Definition and Classification of Learning Disorders

Consistent with most discussions of learning problems, DSM-5 defines a Learning Disorder as "persistent difficulties learning keystone academic skills (Criterion A), with onset during the years of formal schooling (i.e., the developmental period)" (p. 68). DSM-5 allows for diagnosis based on deficits in the broad categories of reading, mathematics, and written expression, as well as the specific skills of reading rate, fluency, comprehension, spelling, and accuracy and fluency in calculations. Specific Learning Disorder is one of the few categories for which psychological testing is explicitly considered. There remain, however, many unresolved issues in how to operationalize the concept of a Learning Disorder. This is the central conflict in efforts to delineate the boundaries of learning problems. Poor school performance can arise from a multitude of influences. A Mental Disorder per se is neither necessary nor sufficient to explain school failure. In addition to this enduring puzzle, ongoing research continues to challenge traditional ideas about learning problems (see, e.g., Colker, Shaywitz, Shaywitz, & Simon, 2014; Shaywitz, Escobar, Shaywitz, Fletcher, & Makuch, 1990; Shaywitz, Shaywitz, Fletcher, & Escobar, 1990).

Consistent with the IDEA definition of specific learning disability, DSM-5 includes language encouraging the examiner to ensure that the symptoms are not better explained by intellectual disabilities, sensory deficits, other mental or neurological disorders, language proficiency, lack of educational experience, and other psychosocial variables when diagnosing Specific Learning Disorder. Specific Learning Disorder and Intellectual Disability may be diagnosed concurrently, but the practical applications of concurrent diagnoses of Intellectual Disability and a Learning Disorder are limited; only special cases (e.g., Mild Intellectual Disability and a very severe and focused Specific Learning Disorder) are likely to qualify. The conceptual implications are, however, significant. The Specific Learning Disorder diagnosis in DSM-5 is written in a much more flexible manner than in previous editions, with a corresponding increase in the examiner's responsibility to assess each individual case carefully. The next DSM-IV-TR note provides a detailed discussion of the changes in the diagnosis of learning problems from the last edition of the DSM.

Three specifiers for Specific Learning Disorders in DSM-5 reflect the primary academic areas of difficulty, although a specifier is not required. These specifiers allow the examiner to designate any and all impaired academic areas. The three main specifiers are With Impairment in Reading, With Impairment in Written Expression, and With Impairment in Mathematics. In cases in which more than one specifier applies, all should be included. For example, a child may receive the diagnosis of 315.00 (F81.0)

Specific Learning Disorder With Impairment in Reading, With Impairment in Word Reading Accuracy; 315.2 (F81.81) Specific Learning Disorder With Impairment in Written Expression, With Impairment in Spelling Accuracy and Clarity or Organization of Written Expression. (Because individuals often present with more than one area of deficit, we discuss them in more detail under "Associated Problems and Diagnoses," later in the chapter.) For a solid background in the complexities of diagnosing learning disorders, the reader is referred to Flanagan and Alfonso (2010). The IDEA Note on page 59 sets forth how Learning Disorders relate to eligibility for services under IDEA.

DSM-IV-TR Note. Changes in DSM-5 for Specific Learning Disorder

A few major changes are worth noting in regard to the diagnosis of Specific Learning Disorder using DSM-5 relative to DSM-IV-TR. The first noteworthy change is the combination of three separate disorders (i.e., Reading Disorder, Mathematics Disorder, and Disorder of Written Expression) into a singular disorder, Specific Learning Disorder. After providing this diagnosis, the clinician uses specifiers to designate the particular presentation of the disorder (i.e., With Impairment in Reading, Mathematics, or Written Expression), as well as its severity (i.e., Mild, Moderate, or Severe). When more than one impairment is noted, the clinician is to provide specifiers for all affected areas separately. It is important to note that this change is not without its critics (e.g., Colker et al., 2014). Colker and colleagues (2014) provide legal, medical, and scientific evidence against combining dyslexia, or reading disorder, with the other learning disorders. They argue that dyslexia is well established as a learning disorder and should be identified as a separate, exemplar classification, with other "less well defined" learning problems being grouped into a residual diagnosis of "Other Learning Disorders." They also address the potential legal and legislative confusion that may arise from a move away from more specific identification of reading disorders as a unique category. Zumeta, Zirkel, and Danielson (2014) voice similar concerns in a more general way in their review of legislation and legal initiatives in addressing specific learning disabilities. (See related comments in the next Professional Note.) These arguments parallel some of the concerns that have been voiced about the combination of Autistic Disorder, Asperger's Disorder, and Pervasive Developmental Disorder into a single Autism Spectrum Disorder category.

Professional Note. Broader Societal Implications of Mental Health Diagnostic Schemes

Although the authors of DMS-5 present it as a tool for physicians and other mental health professionals and caution against its application in arenas for which it was not designed, the reality is that it will be used in legal, legislative, appropriation, and education decisions, and this reality has perhaps been inadequately attended to in the process of composing the document. Zumeta and colleagues (2014) discuss the far-reaching societal, legal, legislative, and educational consequences of changes in diagnostic categories. Although one can sympathize somewhat with the editors of this edition in that they were charged only with working on a psychiatric classification system for professionals, it is at best naive for them to believe that other agents and agencies in our interconnected world would not be affected by their changes and react, for good or bad, to alterations in categories. These changes will inevitably reverberate in Individualized Education Program (IEP) meetings in schools, federal and state legislative appropriation committees, units charged with addressing the disabilities of students at colleges and universities, and courtrooms in which civil and criminal cases are being adjudicated. What the appropriate balance between mental health professionals and other "stakeholders" in the process should be in future revisions is a question without an easy answer, but perhaps the process of arriving at the next answer should be as clear and public as possible.

Another major change in this category is a shift from focusing on standardized test scores in DSM-IV-TR to a more comprehensive evaluation of all available data. A shift in the language in the diagnostic criteria also reflects an expectation of adopting a response-to-intervention approach: It reads " . . . symptoms that have persisted for at least 6 months, *despite the provision of interventions that target those difficulties*" (p. 66, emphasis added). For example, the diagnosis of Reading Disorder using DSM-IV-TR required a discrepancy between reading achievement and age, cognitive ability, and education, as measured by standardized tests. Diagnosis of Specific Learning Disorder with Impairment in Reading using DSM-5 requires at least one symptom of reading difficulty (e.g., reading fluency or reading comprehension) that places the individual's performance significantly below expectations or interferes with daily functioning, as demonstrated by integration of all information, including developmental and academic history, school reports, and comprehensive assessment or a documented history of impairment for those over 17 years of age. With DSM-5, learning difficulties must begin while the individual is of school age. DSM-5 is also more comprehensive in providing a list of rule-outs, and these rule-outs are conveniently consistent with those used for IDEA classification (e.g., adequate educational opportunity, lack of language proficiency for instruction).

Finally, the Specific Learning Disorder diagnosis requires one or more of six possible symptoms. This list of six includes "difficulties with spelling" independently from other deficits in reading and/or writing. What was formerly 315.9 Learning Disorder Not Otherwise Specified does not appear in DSM-5; however, with the allowance for a deficit in a single academic skill to qualify for a Specific Learning Disorder diagnosis, it is possible to capture these individuals. Thus diagnosis of cases that would have been labeled Learning Disorder Not Otherwise Specified under DSM-IV-TR will need to be treated in a different way under DSM-5. Examiners will need to determine specific impaired subskills, even if they are unable to identify a specific academic domain or broader area of deficit. Even in the absence of an identified broad area of deficit (e.g., with impairment in reading), the diagnosis of Specific Learning Disorder should reflect the basic concept of a Learning Disorder; that is, it should involve academic difficulty and failure that cannot be better accounted for by a low level of general intellectual functioning, inadequate effort, low subcultural valuation of school achievement, or the expected disruption of life caused by many mental disorders (especially Disruptive Behavior Disorders, Mood Disorders, Anxiety Disorders, and Psychotic Disorders). There is a real danger that the more socially acceptable diagnostic classification of Specific Learning Disorder will be used when other conceptualizations (Mild Intellectual Disability, Borderline Intellectual Functioning, or Academic Problem—the latter two, of course, are not Mental Disorders) may be more valid. We can only suggest that we are all ultimately best served when diagnostic classification systems (including DSM-5) are used as honestly and as accurately as possible. For a related discussion of the potential pitfalls of these changes, see the Professional Note on pages 57–58.

IDEA Note. Learning Disorders and IDEA

"Specific learning disabilities" are identified qualifying conditions for special education services under IDEA. A Specific Learning Disorder identified in DSM-5 will establish a "specific learning disability" and thus may qualify a child for services under IDEA. Differences between the DSM-5 and IDEA views of learning handicaps may arise, however, out of particular state or district formulations of specific learning disabilities, which often specify a magnitude of discrepancy between measures of aptitude and achievement required to qualify a child for services (e.g., 22 standard score points) or a persistent failure to respond to evidence-based intervention aimed at addressing the deficit in the general education classroom. As we have noted in our text discussion, DSM-5 requires that "the affected academic skills are substantially and quantifiably below those expected for the individual's chronological age, and cause significant interference with academic or occupational performance, or activities of daily living . . . " (p. 67). An exact operational definition of "substantially below" is not given, but DSM-5 requires that a comprehensive assessment be conducted and information from all areas of functioning and the person's history be considered in determining diagnosis. As is always the case in DSM-5, the professional judgment of the examiner is the ultimate deciding factor. Although it is clear that educational classifications are not always decided by a strict adherence to state or district formulations (MacMillan,

Gresham, Siperstein, & Bocian, 1996), a critical difference is that in DSM-5, the decisive role of clinical judgment is seen as justified and desirable (p. 19) and is an individual, not a team, decision, as is the case with special education classification. In short, IDEA's concept of a "specific learning disability" is essentially the same as DSM-5's concept of Specific Learning Disorder, but the boundaries of classification do not always perfectly coincide between the two systems. For example, a boy who is intellectually gifted may qualify for the DSM-5 diagnosis of Specific Learning Disorder, but a school-based team may decide that he does not qualify for special education services under IDEA because this student is performing adequately (e.g., earning Cs) even if he is not performing to his full potential given his intellectual ability.

Academic or Educational Problem

Academic Problem, like Borderline Intellectual Functioning, is a V code. This classification can be used to cover cases of academic problems that are not attributable to a mental disorder—for example, a young person's failing classes in the absence of a Learning or Communication Disorder or any other Mental Disorder that would account for these outcomes. In our experience, the designation of Academic Problem should serve as a cue for further investigation into a child's or adolescent's adjustment, family circumstances, social relationships, and environment. Either abrupt or gradual changes in school performance may be early objective signs of difficulty with the many developmental hurdles of childhood and adolescence (i.e., peer pressures, sexuality, substance use experimentation, lifestyle choices, or the demands of part-time employment on time and energy). Poor school performance is one of the best established risk factors for dropping out of school (Oakland, 1992), and it deserves serious evaluation and aggressive assistance.

Associated Problems and Diagnoses

The linkages between learning problems and other cognitive, behavioral, and emotional characteristics of children are complex and not fully understood—a reality well appreciated by practicing school psychologists. Statistical associations have been reported between Specific Learning Disorders in particular and academic underachievement in general, as well as between Specific Learning Disorders and a number of other major Mental Disorders: Conduct Disorder, Oppositional Defiant Disorder, Attention-Deficit/Hyperactivity Disorder, Major Depressive Disorder, Dysthymic Disorder, and Anxiety Disorders. A history of Developmental Coordination Disorder (see later in the chapter) and/or Communication Disorders may be found in the background of many children with Specific Learning Disorders; these previous difficulties may have largely resolved or may never have been serious enough actually to warrant diagnosis. Finally, meeting the diagnostic criteria for multiple academic domains and/or subskills within the Specific Learning Disorder diagnosis defined in DSM-5 is common in a given child. Indeed, multiple diagnoses are probably the rule rather than the exception.

A good deal of attention has been paid to the social problems of children with learning disabilities. These co-occurring issues may be a significant factor in the morbidity associated with Specific Learning Disorders, especially for the difficulties labeled "nonverbal learning disabilities." The social learning problems of children with Specific Learning Disorders may be one important influence contributing to an elevated risk for personality trait disturbance and Personality Disorders in adults with a childhood history of learning problems (Khan, Cowan, & Roy, 1997). However, as is true of many other topics regarding Specific Learning Disorders, much additional research is needed to understand these relations fully. We are convinced that advances in the empirical and conceptual understanding of Specific Learning Disorders will require examination at the subskill specifier level to reduce this heterogeneous diagnostic grouping, as suggested by some researchers (e.g., Colker et al., 2014).

Comorbidities with and among the Specific Learning Disorders

Reading problems are among the most common academic difficulties encountered in school settings and are certainly the most often investigated. As stated previously, DSM-5 formulation allows examiners to specify deficits in broad academic domains, as well as narrow subskills within these domains. Thus examiners can narrowly identify impairments, including those within the broad domain of reading (e.g., reading fluency, reading comprehension), as well as other deficits. There are strong associations between Specific Learning Disorder with Impairment in Reading and problems with phonological processing, and a history (not necessarily current) of Speech Sound Disorder (formerly Phonological Disorder under DSM-IV-TR) may be found. Frequent comorbid associations with the other two academic domain specifiers within Specific Learning Disorder are noted. Specific Learning Disorder with Impairment in Reading also shows associations with other Mental Disorders, especially Attention-Deficit/Hyperactivity Disorder, Communication Disorders, Developmental Coordination Disorder, Autism Spectrum Disorder, Disruptive Behavior Disorders, and (in older children or adolescents) Mood Disorders and Substance Use Disorders. Untangling the nature, direction, and causality of these associations is an ongoing task and may be complicated by gender-specific pathways (Frick et al., 1991; Shaywitz, Shaywitz, et al., 1990; Smart, Sanson, & Prior, 1996).

Specific Learning Disorder with Impairment in Mathematics and Specific Learning Disorder with Impairment in Written Expression are provided in DSM-5 as additional specifiers of learning problems. Although clinical experience suggests that learning disability confined to arithmetic skills does occur among children and adolescents, the unique occurrence of writing problems is less clearly established. Problems of written expression usually occur in association with reading problems. A given child may actually meet criteria for all three of the major domain specifiers in DSM-5, with significant impairments noted in reading, written expression, and mathematics.

The text of DSM-5 acknowledges that less is known about Specific Learning Disorders with impairments in written expression and those with impairments in mathematics relative to those with impairments in reading. One fine point is worth noting: Poor handwriting alone is not diagnosed as Specific Learning Disorder with Impairment in Written Expression. In contrast, poor spelling is now a sole symptom that qualifies for a Specific Learning Disorder diagnosis under DSM-5, although it usually occurs along with reading deficits, except for the interesting and unusual cases of isolated spelling disability with good reading skills (so-called "benign spelling dyspraxia"). Poor handwriting may be a symptom of Developmental Coordination Disorder (see later in the chapter). The boundaries between these various categories are conceptually problematic, and diagnosis of the individual child will ultimately require the examiner's best judgment as to the diagnosis or combination of diagnoses that most meaningfully and fully captures the essential features of a particular young person's difficulties.

COMMUNICATION DISORDERS

Also included in the "Neurodevelopmental" chapter are the Communication Disorders. This section covers several language and speech problems often found in youth: Language Disorder, Speech Sound Disorder, Childhood-Onset Fluency Disorder (Stuttering), Social (Pragmatic) Communication Disorder, and Unspecified Communication Disorder. Although it was written in the era of DSM-IV, a good introduction to this specialty area for the school and child clinical psychologist is Cohen's (2001) text. A still older reference, Cantwell and Baker (1987), continues to have relevance to this topic. Language—the capacity to represent, manipulate, and communicate

IDEA Note. Communication Disorders and IDEA

Speech or language impairments are identified qualifying conditions for special education services under IDEA. Communication Disorders as defined by DSM-5 typically equate with speech or language deficits as identified by IDEA, although it is possible that a particular state or school district may formulate more specific operational definitions of a speech or language impairment that are more restrictive than the criteria in DSM-5 (cf. the IDEA Note on pp. 59–60).

ideas symbolically—is one of the most complex productions of the human brain. Oral speech is one of the major vehicles for this symbolic communication in most individuals. Communication difficulties can be disruptive of typical development, and the categorization within DSM-5 appears crude at best (see the American Speech–Language–Hearing Association [ASHA], 2012, recommended revisions to DSM-5). School psychologists are well prepared to assess several of aspects of communication difficulties (Bray, Kehle, & Theodore, 2014) to inform intervention. Beyond assessment and assistance with behavioral intervention, collaboration with a qualified speech/language therapist is advised. The next IDEA Note sets forth how the Communication Disorders relate to eligibility for services under IDEA.

Communication Disorders have been associated with Specific Learning Disabilities and with cognitive problems. The linkage between reading problems and an earlier history of articulation or language problems has been discussed previously. Communication Disorders can also be sequelae of traumatic brain injury in children (Cahill, Murdoch, & Theodoros, 2005; Jordan, Murdoch, Buttsworth, & Hudson-Tennent, 1995; Jordan, Ozanne, & Murdoch, 1990). In children, a transient "acquired aphasia" may be associated with a general medical condition such as encephalitis or traumatic brain injury. If the language disruption persists beyond the acute recovery period for the general medical condition, then a diagnosis of a Communication Disorder becomes appropriate. Communication Disorders secondary to traumatic brain injury may persist over extended periods and have important implications for academic and social adjustment. A younger age at the time of injury and greater severity of injury are both associated with poorer outcome (Ewing-Cobbs, Miner, Fletcher, & Levin, 1989; Jordan, Ozanne, & Murdoch, 1988; Yorkston, Jaffe, Polissar, Liao, & Fay, 1997). Communication Disorders secondary to traumatic brain injury may involve both oral and written language production (Yorkston et al., 1997), and an associated diagnosis of Specific Learning Disability with Impairments in Written Expression may be warranted. (Traumatic brain injury is discussed further in the "Major and Mild Neurocognitive Disorder" section in Chapter 5 of this book.)

DSM-5 identified one language problem, Language Disorder; two speech problems, Speech Sound Disorder and Childhood-Onset Fluency Disorder; a new communication disorder, Social Communication Disorder, which could also be construed as a language disorder; and a category for residual cases, Unspecified Communication Disorder.

The Language Disorder category subsumes the two language disorder categories of DSM-IV: Expressive Language Disorder and Mixed Expressive and Receptive Language Disorder. The absence of specifiers for expressive and receptive–expressive subtypes seems puzzling given the research literature on this topic. The new category of Social (Pragmatic) Communication Disorder appears to be another language disorder that focuses on difficulties in social communication. Both of these disorders are differentiated from Autism Spectrum Disorders (in which communication impairments are a defining feature) by the absence of stereotyped actions and constriction of age-typical repertoires of behavior. In both cases, the communication deficits must exceed what would be expected in terms of any intellectual disability or sensory or motor deficits.

Two speech disorders are included in DSM-5. The first is Speech Sound Disorder, which was previously labeled Phonological Disorder (DSM-IV) and, previous to that, Developmental Articulation Disorder (DSM-III). The basic character of the problem, difficulty with the production of speech phonemes, is unchanged. The second is Childhood-Onset Fluency Disorder (Stuttering), previously referred to as Stuttering. There is no discussion of other common speech problems, such as difficulty with amplitude, voice, or delayed speech. The definitions of both Speech Sound Disorder and Childhood-Onset Fluency Disorder (Stuttering) are typical of discussions within the field of speech pathology. Speech problems may be diagnosed concurrently with Intellectual Disability or with neurological disorders involving sensory or speech–motor deficit if the speech disturbance is greater than could be reasonably accounted for by the comorbid condition. Speech Sound Disorder will be of interest to many school psychologists because a history of articulation difficulties is common in some cases of reading disorders and other learning disabilities (as noted earlier) and may help identify a phonological processing pattern of reading disability. Articulation problems, which often improve or resolve with age, are associated with a variety of concurrent developmental problems (Namasivayam et al., 2013).

The category of Unspecified Communication Disorder covers language and speech disorders that cause distress or impairment and that are not captured by the four formal diagnoses of the sections. Given the range of speech and language problems identified by specialists in this field that are not formally classified by DSM-5—voice disorders, developmental dysarthrias, primary developmental anomia, and other phenomena targeted by speech and language pathologists—this residual category will be a heterogeneous group of limited use for anything beyond the crudest record keeping. Speech and language problems graduate into areas in which psychologists have limited training or expertise, yet the expertise of school psychologists allows for the assessment of and behavioral intervention for Communication Disorders (Bray et al., 2014).

Finally, it may be worth mentioning Selective Mutism (discussed in Chapter 9) briefly here because it is sometimes thought of as a communication problem. However, DSM-5 does not group it with the Communication Disorders. It is placed in the "Anxiety Disorders" chapter. This placement change began in DSM-IV and reflects the current understanding of Selective Mutism as a manifestation of underlying anxiety (Dummit et al., 1997; Keeton & Budinger, 2012). Only about one-third of children with Selective Mutism have a history of other speech or language problems (Steinhausen & Juzi, 1996).

MOTOR DISORDERS

Developmental Coordination Disorder

Developmental Coordination Disorder is the first entry in the Motor Disorders section of the Neurodevelopmental Disorders chapter of DSM-5. The other disorders in this section include Stereotypic Movement Disorder, Tic Disorders, Other Specified Tic Disorder, and Unspecified Tic Disorder. Developmental Coordination Disorder is identified as impairment in the development of motor coordination that interferes significantly with scholastic achievement or general daily activities, including play. The disorder category is not due to a general medical condition, including visual impairment. It can be made together with a diagnosis of Intellectual Disability, but the degree of motor incoordination must be greater than that which would be expected as an associated feature of the Intellectual Disability. Similarly, it can be made together with a diagnosis of Autism Spectrum Disorder, but the degree of motor incoordination must be greater than that which would be expected as an associated feature of the Autism Spectrum Disorder. This disorder can also be diagnosed concurrently with Attention-Deficit/Hyperactivity Disorder. It is discussed here, however, because of its particularly close association with the Learning Disorders. The IDEA Note on pages 66–67 sets forth how this disorder relates to eligibility for services under IDEA.

Developmental Coordination Disorder was introduced in DSM-III-R to facilitate research into the possible links between various aspects of development and learning and behavior problems. Some clinicians have treated nonspecific motor incoordination as a "soft" or "minor" neurological sign. For a detailed discussion of changes from the last edition of DSM in this diagnostic category, see the next DSM-IV-TR Note. There is little empirical literature on this DSM diagnosis, and it is probably too soon to know how useful it will prove. Related concepts, however, have been studied and found to be associated with academic difficulties. Fletcher-Flinn, Elmes, and Strugnell (1997) reported on a group of 30 children in New Zealand diagnosed with "congenital developmental coordination disorder" and found that 25% had severe reading difficulties and 30% severe spelling disabilities. The spelling problems were associated with visual discrimination, but the reading difficulties were not; phonological awareness and spelling problems were associated with reading difficulties. Associations between motor control and clumsiness, visual–spatial perception, and attention problems continue to be investigated (Hellgren, Gillberg, Bahenholm, & Gillberg, 1994; Henderson, Barnett, & Henderson, 1994).

DSM-IV-TR Note. Changes in DSM-5 for Developmental Coordination Disorder

The criteria for Developmental Coordination Disorder have not changed a great deal from DSM-IV-TR to DSM-5. The main changes are the addition of criteria C, that onset must occur "during the developmental period," (p. 74) and the description of rule-outs in the criteria. DSM-5 requires that the motor deficits not be better explained by intellectual disability, visual impairment, or other medical condition that may affect motor ability (e.g., cerebral palsy). The DSM-5 criteria also specifically include the acquisition and execution of motor skills, not simply the performance of daily activities that require motor functioning, as the DSM-IV-TR did.

IDEA Note. Developmental Coordination Disorder and IDEA

A DSM-5 diagnosis of Developmental Coordination Disorder can form the basis for a qualification of a child as eligible for special services under IDEA through the other health impairment category if the disorder adversely affects the child's educational performance. The functional impairment criterion for the category will have special significance if this diagnosis is being used to qualify inclusion under IDEA: "The motor skills deficit in Criterion A significantly and persistently interferes with activities of daily living appropriate to chronological age (e.g., self-care and self-maintenance) and impacts academic/school productivity . . . " (p. 74).

We have found the phenomenon indexed by the diagnosis of Developmental Coordination Disorder in several children and adolescents with learning problems, especially those who fit the so-called "nonverbal learning disability" pattern. We suggest careful evaluation of Developmental Coordination Disorder as a possible comorbid diagnosis in children diagnosed with Specific Learning Disorder with impairment in mathematics, which has also been linked by Rourke (1989) to his concept of nonverbal learning disabilities. Increased awareness of this category should lead to a better understanding of the links among sensory, motor, cognitive, and academic development in children. In our clinical experience, a comorbid diagnosis of Specific Learning Disorder has helped in eligibility decisions for special education services under the Specific Learning Disability and Other Health Impaired categories, though eligibility for either qualifies a child for the full umbrella of relevant special education services.

Tic Disorders

Five diagnoses are provided for the classification of Tic Disorders: Tourette's Disorder, Persistent (Chronic) Motor or Vocal Tic Disorder, Provisional Tic Disorder, Other Specified Tic Disorder, and Unspecified Tic Disorder. Broadly described, these categories represent various combinations of tic pattern (vocal and/or motor) and duration (less than or more than 1 year). All but the last two categories (i.e., Other Specified Tic Disorder and Unspecified Tic Disorder) require an onset prior to 18 years of age. Tourette's Disorder involves both motor and vocal tics and a prolonged duration; Persistent (Chronic) Motor or Vocal Tic Disorder reflects either motor or vocal tics and a prolonged duration; Provisional Tic Disorder covers any pattern that has caused difficulty for less than a year; Other Specified Tic Disorder covers significant problems that interfere with functioning but do not meet the diagnostic criteria for the other categories (e.g., onset after the age of 18), and Unspecified Tic Disorder is used when the clinician notes the presence of these symptoms but chooses not to indicate why the criteria for another tic disorder are not met, perhaps because insufficient information is available. A great deal of psychological interest has focused on Tourette's Disorder and on the possibility of a spectrum of neurobehavioral disorders that includes many Tic Disorders, Obsessive–Compulsive Disorder, and Attention-Deficit/Hyperactivity Disorder. There are significant comorbidities between Tourette's Disorder and Obsessive–Compulsive Disorder, as well as between Tourette's Disorder and Attention-Deficit/Hyperactivity Disorder. Walter and Carter (1997) suggest that learning problems are also overrepresented in children with Tourette's Disorder, although most do not have learning or cognitive disabilities. Children who present with Tic Disorders should be periodically evaluated for attention-deficit problems, as well as anxiety symptoms, especially obsessive–compulsive patterns.

Stereotypic Movement Disorder

Stereotypic Movement Disorder (Atypical Stereotyped Movement Disorder in DSM-III, Stereotypy/Habit Disorder in DSM-III-R) consists of repetitive, nonpurposeful motor movements that have a "driven" quality. The actions may be self-injurious, in which case the specifier With Self-Injurious Behavior is added to the diagnosis. If the behavior is associated with a known genetic or medical condition, that condition should also be specified. This type of behavior is a common associated feature of Autism Spectrum Disorders. Stereotypic Movement Disorder may also be associated with Intellectual Disability. This diagnosis can be made concurrently with that of Intellectual Disability or Autism Spectrum Disorder if the stereotypic or self-injurious actions are problematic enough to warrant a treatment focus.

7

Highly Atypical Symptom Patterns

Autism Spectrum Disorders and Psychoses

OVERVIEW

The conceptualization of the most severe behavioral disorders in DSM-5 reflects the interaction of two considerations: (1) the appearance of qualitatively distinctive and disruptive signs and symptoms (e.g., psychotic symptoms, significant behavior deficits, stereotyped self-stimulation) and (2) temporal features of the disturbance (age of onset, duration). Autism Spectrum Disorders involve major disruptions in various aspects of typical development—reciprocal social responsiveness, communication, an increasingly complex behavioral repertoire—as well as an onset early in life, either with or without a preceding period of typical development. The Psychotic Disorders involve characteristic symptoms (i.e., delusions, hallucinations, profound disorganization of behavior, negative symptoms) occurring over various periods of time (less than a month, 1–6 months, more than 6 months). These two groupings (plus a few other disorders in which psychotic symptoms may appear) represent the most recent attempts to define some of the most severe and puzzling disturbances of behavior and adjustment seen in human beings. Research continues, and it is doubtful that DSM-5 will represent the last word on marking the boundaries of the Autism Spectrum Disorders and the Psychotic Disorders; nevertheless, the formulations of DSM-5 appear to constitute both an advance over previous editions of DSM and a basis for reasonably objective and reliable evaluation.

AUTISM SPECTRUM DISORDERS

The occurrence of severe disorders in childhood associated not only with the behavioral deficits evident in Intellectual Disability but also with highly unusual behavioral excesses or "deviant" behavior has been recognized for some time. Labels such as "childhood psychosis" and "childhood schizophrenia" were formally applied to such children, often in such an all-inclusive and noncritical manner that little meaning was conveyed (see, e.g., Creak, 1961, 1963). The current definition of these disorders as Autism Spectrum Disorders both highlights their essential features (multiple impairment in major areas of development and onset early in life) and helps differentiate these psychopathologies from the common forms of psychosis disorder seen in adolescents and adults. An important change in DSM-5 from its predecessor is the integration of several diagnostic categories into one inclusive diagnosis. This change, on the surface, appears to be a reversal of the divisions that were made in DSM-IV from the categories in DSM-III-R; however, this change reflects a deeper recognition that Autism Spectrum Disorders present on a continuum of functioning. Thus, the current diagnostic criteria allow the examiner to identify specifiers that help to characterize an individual's presentation on the autism spectrum. That is, what was formerly covered in four diagnostic categories in DSM-IV-TR is now captured in one diagnosis. The next DSM-IV-TR Note describes the changes in the classification of Autism Spectrum Disorders from DSM-IV-TR to DSM-5, and the next IDEA Note sets forth how Autism Spectrum Disorders relate to eligibility for services under IDEA.

DSM-IV-TR Note. From Five to One Autism Spectrum Disorder

The category of Autism Spectrum Disorder is one of the biggest changes from DSM-IV-TR to DSM-5. What was formerly covered in four diagnostic categories (i.e., Autistic Disorder, Rett's Disorder, Asperger's Disorder, and Pervasive Developmental Disorder Not Otherwise Specified) is now covered in one diagnostic category: Autism Spectrum Disorder. These other categories are no longer listed as separate disorders in DSM-5. With the exception of Childhood Disintegrative Disorder, which was completely removed from DSM-5, practitioners are directed to assign a diagnosis of Autism Spectrum Disorder for these cases. For example, children formerly diagnosed with Rett's Disorder under DSM-IV would receive the DSM-5 diagnosis of Autism Spectrum Disorder associated with Rett syndrome. In cases in which only social communication deficits are noted in the absence of a limited range of interests, behaviors, and activities, examiners are advised to consider the appropriateness of a Social (Pragmatic) Communication Disorder diagnosis.

IDEA Note. Autism Spectrum Disorders and IDEA

According to the U.S. Department of Education's IDEA 2004 website (*www.gpo.gov/fdsys/pkg/PLAW-108publ446/html/PLAW-108publ446.htm*), "Autism" has been defined as follows:

(i) Autism means a developmental disability significantly affecting verbal and nonverbal communication and social interaction, generally evident before age three, that adversely affects a child's educational performance. Other characteristics often associated with autism are engagement in repetitive activities and stereotyped movements, resistance to environmental change or change in daily routines, and unusual responses to sensory experiences.
(ii) Autism does not apply if a child's educational performance is adversely affected primarily because the child has an emotional disturbance, as defined in paragraph (c)(4) of this section.
(iii) A child who manifests the characteristics of autism after age three could be identified as having autism if the criteria in paragraph (c)(1)(i) of this section are satisfied.

The DSM-5 diagnostic criteria for Autism Spectrum Disorder more closely align with the IDEA definition of Autism than did its predecessor. That is, the diagnostic category of Autism Spectrum Disorder subsumes what were previously four distinct disorders (i.e., Autistic Disorder, Rett's Disorder, Asperger's Disorder, and Pervasive Developmental Disorder Not Otherwise Specified) that were considered for eligibility under the more generic IDEA category of "autism." As discussed previously, the single DSM-5 category for Autism Spectrum Disorder reflects a continuum of impairment, with those demonstrating greater impairment being more likely to qualify for special education services under IDEA. An important key to determination is likely the extent to which the disorder affects the child's educational performance. The use of specifiers for comorbid disorders and severity will likely assist in documenting the extent of a child's impairment, including its influence on academic functioning. In our experiences, often children presenting with Autism Spectrum Disorder are deemed eligible for accommodations under 504 or special education services under IDEA. In some cases, children who fall on the higher functioning end of the spectrum but do not meet the criteria under the autism category can qualify relatively easily for services under IDEA because of the severity of functional impairment seen in children afflicted with these global disturbances of adjustment. Either the "emotional disturbance" category of Part B or the "other health impairment" category can be used to document the handicaps for academic, social, and personal adjustment in these cases.

Additional Diagnoses to Be Considered

Mental Retardation occurs in up to 75–80% of children diagnosed with Autism Spectrum Disorder and carries important prognostic significance. If a child's general intellectual functioning is compromised to a significant degree (IQ less than 70), the additional diagnosis of Intellectual Disability is made. Neurological problems associated with Autism Spectrum Disorder include seizure disorders, which usually develop in adolescence. There is an association between Intellectual Disability and seizure disorder development in children with Autism Spectrum Disorder, and both are associated with a poorer prognosis (Morgan, 1990).

Precluded Diagnoses

Stereotyped, nonpurposeful motor movements (self-stimulation) are also characteristic of children with Autism Spectrum Disorder. The work of Lovaas suggests that these responses are not benign; especially at high frequencies, they actively compete against most appropriate learning (Lovaas, Newsom, & Hickman, 1987). Stereotyped movements are a symptom of Autism Spectrum Disorder, but it is only diagnosed simultaneously if it results in self-injurious behavior that becomes an independent focus of treatment. Various other diagnoses (e.g., Developmental Coordination Disorder, the Communication Disorders, Pica, Rumination Disorder, Selective Mutism, Reactive Attachment Disorder) are also precluded under the general hierarchical arrangement of DSM categories, in which more pervasive categories subsume more specific diagnoses (in most cases).

PSYCHOSES

A second group of diagnoses that an examiner should consider when confronted with severely disturbed and disorganized maladjustment in a child or adolescent are those that have traditionally been subsumed under the heading of "psychoses." This chapter includes diagnostic criteria for Delusional Disorder, Psychotic Disorder, Schizophreniform Disorder, Schizophrenia, Schizoaffective Disorder, Substance/Medication-Induced Psychotic Disorder, Brief Psychotic Disorder Due to Another Medical Condition, Catatonia Associated with Another Mental Disorder (Catatonia Specifier), Catatonic Disorder Due to Another Medical Condition, Unspecified Catatonia, Other Specified Schizophrenic Spectrum and Other Psychotic Disorder, and Unspecified Schizophrenic Spectrum and Other Psychotic Disorder. The introduction to the "Schizophrenia Spectrum and Other Psychotic Disorders" chapter of DSM-5 provides definitions of symptoms relevant to this domain and a brief discussion of how to approach diagnosis within this category. That is, it directs examiners to rule out lesser disorders (e.g., Delusional Disorder) and those that are time limited (e.g., Brief Psychotic Disorder) before considering the more severe diagnostic categories (e.g., Schizophrenia). These changes are detailed in the next DSM-IV-TR Note. We discuss Psychotic Disorders next, along with a few other disorders in which psychotic symptoms may appear. The next IDEA Note sets forth how the Psychotic Disorders relate to eligibility for services under IDEA.

IDEA Note. Psychotic Disorders

Schizophrenia and other Psychotic Disorders in DSM-5 can certainly qualify for inclusion under the "Emotional Disturbance" category of IDEA. A Psychotic Disorder exemplifies the basic meaning of a serious emotional disturbance, both for the general public and for members of professional disciplines involved with mental health. The disruptive symptoms and devastating life consequences of Schizophrenia and the other Psychotic Disorders easily fulfill the requirements for a handicapping condition in the IDEA legislation.

DSM-IV-TR Note. Changes in DSM-5 for Schizophrenia

The diagnostic criteria for Schizophrenia have not changed much from DSM-IV-TR to DSM-5. One change is a requirement that at least one of three positive symptoms is present: delusions, hallucinations, or disorganized speech. DSM-IV-TR also included five subtypes of Schizophrenia (Paranoid, Disorganized, Catatonic, Undifferentiated, and Residual Types), but these do not appear in DSM-5. Finally, the specifiers are slightly different between these two editions. DSM-5 prompts the examiner to indicate whether the individual is experiencing his or her first episode or multiple episodes and whether the individual is currently fulfilling the criteria (i.e., acute), is improving but still meets some of the criteria (i.e., in partial remission), or met the criteria in the past but does not currently meet them (i.e., full remission). For example, someone experiencing a first active episode may be given the diagnosis of Schizophrenia, first episode, currently in acute episode. Examiners are also to indicate the presence of catatonia when appropriate and specify severity (i.e., Mild, Moderate, Severe).

Schizophrenia

The core syndrome definition in this chapter of DSM-5 is that of Schizophrenia. Schizophrenia has been the paradigm psychotic disorder since Kraepelin's original discussion of "dementia praecox" and Bleuler's elaboration of the primary and secondary symptoms of "the schizophrenias."

Schizophrenia is defined by a group of characteristic symptoms that have persisted over at least 1 month, with some continuous signs of disturbance for at least 6 months. The DSM-5 Criterion A symptom set contains both positive and negative symptoms. The DSM-5 positive symptoms (four of the five symptoms) are delusions, hallucinations, disorganized speech, and extremely disorganized or catatonic behavior. At least one of the first three positive symptoms must be present for diagnosis. The set of negative symptoms—that is, flattening of mood, impoverished thinking, and problems with goal-directed activities—makes up the fifth criterion symptom. Depressed mood is sometimes discussed as a negative symptom, but in DSM-5 it is included only as an associated symptom. A fuller discussion of negative symptoms would have been helpful; Carpenter, Heinrichs, and Wagman (1988) provide an informative discussion of these symptoms. Additional requirements for the diagnosis of Schizophrenia include a decline in level of general adjustment (or failure to make expected developmental advances, in children and adolescents); an exclusion of Schizoaffective Disorder and of a Mood Disorder with Psychotic Features as explanations for the problematic behaviors; and an exclusion of general medical conditions or substance use effects as the cause of the disorder. As discussed in the last DSM-IV-TR Note on the previous page, the subtypes of Schizophrenia were removed in DSM-5 because of concerns regarding their validity.

There is no unique set of symptoms for childhood- or adolescence-onset Schizophrenia; the same criteria set is used for all ages. Schizophrenia usually shows an initial episode in late adolescence or early adulthood, but childhood-onset cases and early-adolescence-onset cases have been documented and can be diagnosed with the Schizophrenia criteria set (Asarnow, 1994). Werry (1996) has suggested the terms "early onset" for Schizophrenia that develops in childhood or adolescence and "very early onset" for Schizophrenia that develops before age 13; it is useful to be aware of these ideas, but DSM-5 makes no such distinctions. There are developmental features evident in childhood-onset Schizophrenia: An insidious onset is typical; there is usually a history of poor adjustment and speech and language problems in early childhood; and positive symptoms begin to manifest themselves only after the child reaches 6–9 years of age (Asarnow, 2013). About two-thirds of children who are diagnosed with Schizophrenia will also meet criteria for other Mental Disorders (Russell, Bott, & Sammons, 1989). The most common comorbid diagnoses with childhood-onset Schizophrenia are Disruptive Behavior Disorders (Conduct Disorder and Oppositional Defiant Disorder) and Depressive Disorders (Asarnow, 2013). A careful review and consideration of possible alternative explanations should precede any application of this most serious diagnosis to a young person, but there are absolutely cases in which it is indicated.

A major differential diagnosis challenge for early-onset Schizophrenia is Bipolar I Disorder. Werry (1996) suggests that Bipolar I Disorder was probably underdiagnosed in adolescents in the past and may be overdiagnosed currently in youth who show clear evidence of psychotic symptomatology. Based on his long-term follow-up studies of both disorders in children and adolescents, Werry (p. 33) suggests the following indications favoring Schizophrenia as the more likely diagnosis: (1) long-standing premorbid abnormality, (2) psychosis lasting more than 3 months, (3) a deteriorating course, and (4) a family history of Schizophrenia. Werry cautions, however, that long-term follow-up is the only basis upon which to reach a firm conclusion and advises examiners to be willing to reconsider their initial formulations in the light of additional evidence. This is sage advice with respect to all diagnostic activity with youth.

Schizophrenia can be diagnosed concurrently with Autism Spectrum Disorder or in an individual with a history of Autism Spectrum Disorder. The explicit requirement in these cases is that the symptom picture must include prominent delusions or hallucinations. It appears that the co-occurrence of Schizophrenia in children with a history of Autism Spectrum Disorder is no greater than would be expected by chance (Asarnow, 2013). The boundaries and relations between Schizophrenia, Mood Disorders, Autism Spectrum Disorders, and other mental disorders remain an area of active investigation with advances in genetic and brain studies ongoing.

Differentiating psychotic hallucinations from other phenomena in children can be clinically challenging. Pilowsky (1986) has offered some guidelines for evaluating apparent hallucinatory behavior in children. He suggests several aspects of a case that may increase the evaluator's confidence that the child is actually experiencing perceptual distortions: (1) a spontaneous report of hallucinations (vs. material elicited by questioning); (2) vivid hallucinations (vs. reports of vague or indistinct experiences); (3) the child's belief in the reality of the hallucination (vs. reservation and doubt about the nature of the experience); (4) the child's experience that the perceptions are coming from outside the child (vs. the belief that the experiences arise from within the child himself or herself); and (5) the apparent absence of volitional control over the perceptions (vs. the ability to dismiss the voices at will). The empirical literature on hallucinations in children is limited. Our own experiences are that Pilowsky's characteristics may have more positive predictive power than negative predictive power. That is, the presence of the variables he believes to be associated with true hallucinations seems much more informative than their absence does. Hallucinations in children need to be distinguished from a number of normal phenomena

(Pilowsky, 1986): eidetic imagery (total visual recall is much more frequent in children than in adolescents or adults), imaginary companions, and hypnogogic and hypnopompic hallucinations (vivid but normal hallucinations that occur when a child is falling asleep or just waking up).

The evaluation of both hallucinations and delusions in children depends, in part, on the children's ability to distinguish reality from imagination, fantasy, and dream. This distinction becomes increasingly suspect if a child's mental age is less than about 6 years, and diagnostic caution is appropriate. We reiterate Pilowsky's caution regarding spontaneous versus elicited reports of hallucinations in children: Most children are highly suggestible to communications from most adults under many conditions. It is an empirical finding that has been robustly supported. It has been our experiences with over two decades of graduate students that most examiners are relatively unaware of how leading their questions may be. In short, evaluators should regard elicited reports of hallucinations in young children with a healthy suspiciousness in the absence of supporting evidence.

Schizophreniform Disorder

Schizophreniform Disorder is identical to Schizophrenia except for the duration of symptoms. It is, by definition, a disorder of more than 1 month but less than 6 months that meets the criterion set for Schizophrenia. The next Coding Note discusses the duration requirement for Schizophreniform Disorder in more detail.

Brief Psychotic Disorder

Brief Psychotic Disorder is defined as a brief and limited period (1 day to 1 month) of at least one of three positive symptom of psychosis: delusions, hallucinations, and disorganized speech. Extremely disorganized or catatonic behavior may also be present, but it alone does not qualify an individual for this diagnosis. The specifier With Marked Stressor(s) is available, but a major stressor is not required for the diagnosis. With Postpartum Onset is also available as a specifier. The diagnosis of Brief Psychotic Disorder is not made if the symptoms are better accounted for by a Mood Disorder. Careful evaluation is necessary to exclude psychotic symptoms resulting from general medical conditions or use of a substance (medication, toxin, or drug of abuse).

Schizoaffective Disorder

Schizoaffective Disorder reflects a disturbance that concurrently meets the criteria both for Schizophrenia and for a Major Depressive, Manic,

Coding Note. Schizophreniform Disorder in Children and Adolescents

If a young person who shows symptoms meeting the criterion set for Schizophrenia (except for duration of symptoms) recovers in less than 6 months, then the correct diagnosis is Schizophreniform Disorder. If the young person does not recover but 6 months have not yet passed, then the correct diagnosis is Schizophreniform Disorder (Provisional). If the disorder persists longer than 6 months, the diagnosis should be changed to Schizophrenia. The course and duration of the disturbance are critical diagnostic elements in assigning the correct DSM-5 diagnosis for a Psychotic Disorder.

The major difference among Brief Psychotic Disorder, Schizophreniform Disorder, and Schizophrenia involves duration of disturbance: 1 day to 1 month, 1 month to 6 months, and more than 6 months, respectively.

or Mixed Episode of mood symptoms. This can be a confusing diagnostic category, both conceptually and in actual practice. Mood symptoms, especially depression and anhedonia, are common associated symptoms in individuals with Schizophrenia or another Psychotic Disorder. Furthermore, pure mood disorders (both Major Depressive Disorder and Bipolar I and II Disorders) can exacerbate to the point of psychosis (see "Additional Diagnostic Categories Involving Psychosis," later in the chapter). The diagnosis of Schizoaffective Disorder, however, is not made in cases involving isolated symptoms but in cases meeting full criteria for both a Mood Episode (Major Depressive, Manic, or Mixed) and the core symptoms of Schizophrenia simultaneously.

Careful documentation of history is required to establish this diagnosis with any confidence, and this necessity is complicated by the clinical state of an affected individual. That is, young people with Psychotic Disorders are not usually reliable historians. After the psychotic symptoms have begun to clear or respond to treatment, the client may be more responsive to interviewing, but may not remember the information of interest because of the cognitive disruption produced by the psychotic episode. Our experiences have been that only the use of multiple informants who have had regular contact with the individual over the course of his or her problems yields diagnostic confidence with respect to this diagnosis. The next Coding Note presents further reflections on Schizoaffective Disorder.

Delusional Disorder

Delusional Disorder (Paranoia in DSM-III, Delusional [Paranoid] Disorder in DSM-III-R) is a Psychotic Disorder involving prominent delusions

Coding Note. Schizoaffective Disorder in Children and Adolescents

If a child or adolescent concurrently shows full symptoms for both Schizophrenia and a Mood Episode (Major Depressive, Manic, or Mixed), then the correct DSM-5 diagnosis is Schizoaffective Disorder. The boundaries and relations between affective disorders and thought disorders continue to be actively debated and investigated. In our experiences, the clinical population identified with a classification of Schizoaffective Disorder remains highly heterogeneous, with some clients presenting with more Mood Disorder qualities and others with more features of Schizophrenia or other Psychotic Disorders. In DSM-5, this differentiation is captured by the specifiers for Schizoaffective Disorder of "Bipolar type" and "Depressive type." Further work may result in significant revision of the category.

without other prominent symptoms of psychosis. The delusions must be nonbizarre. The individual can have no history of Schizophrenia. This disorder is not usually seen in adolescents or children.

Shared Psychotic Disorder (Folie à Deux)

Shared Psychotic Disorder reflects a delusion that is acquired through a long-standing, intimate relationship with an individual who has a primary Psychotic Disorder with prominent delusions. The special circumstances necessary here obviously limit the prevalence of this possibility, but cases involving children do occur. Children may come to believe and be willing to discuss freely the delusional thoughts of a psychotic parent. The initial contact with such a family may be occasioned by clinical interest in a child or adolescent who has voiced ideas at school that have aroused concern. Only in following up with the family may it become apparent that the young person is merely echoing the beliefs of a parent with a Psychotic Disorder.

This unusual category can raise difficult questions of therapeutic management. In a case one of us saw early in training, a single mother brought her three daughters into a public clinic for vaccinations. The attending resident became concerned over the "crazy ideas" voiced by the two younger girls. When discussing concerns about her daughters with the mother, however, it became apparent that she fully shared (and was probably the origin of) their delusions. An interview with the third and oldest daughter revealed that she too acknowledged the family's unique thoughts but was reticent about sharing these with the examiner; her public behavior appeared to have come under contingency control by the broader community with whom she interacted. The case caused some debate among the professionals involved. The young mother appeared to be clearly delusional and to have taught her children to be delusional; at the same time, this case had only come to our attention because this mother was responsible with respect to the medical needs of her children. (In the city we served, a disturbing percentage of residents had not obtained the recommended health checks and vaccinations for their children.) Furthermore, there was no evidence that the children were neglected or abused. Their medical health was unremarkable. They appeared well fed and clothed, happy and unafraid, positively attached to their caretaker—and delusional. The oldest child showed evidence of having learned to be circumspect about sharing family ideas with outsiders. With the young mother's consent, we communicated with her parents; the parents, we learned, were aware of their daughter's mental health history and communicated regularly with her psychiatrist.

Other Psychotic Disorders

Psychotic Disorder Due to Another Medical Condition and Substance/Medication-Induced Psychotic Disorder reflect psychotic symptoms (delusions and/or hallucinations) associated with specific, established etiologies. Both should be actively evaluated as possibilities in the assessment of acute psychotic symptoms in a young person, especially in the absence of a family history of severe mental health problems. Even in an adolescent with a history of a primary Psychotic Disorder, the possibility of a Substance-Induced Psychotic Disorder should be aggressively considered if there is anything about the circumstances that does not seem consistent with the youth's history. Adolescents, including young people with atypical perceptual processing, are at some risk for substance experimentation. Individuals at risk for Schizophrenia may be especially vulnerable to intense, unpleasant, and/or idiosyncratic reactions to drugs of abuse. Comorbid presentations of Substance Use Disorders and Psychotic Disorders are unfortunately familiar to most mental health workers dealing with adolescents and young adults.

Other Specified Schizophrenia Spectrum and Other Psychotic Disorder (and the diagnosis Unspecified Schizophrenia Spectrum and Other Psychotic Disorder for cases in which the evaluator chooses not to indicate why the criteria were not met) covers a variety of residual cases in which there is evidence of psychotic symptomatology but the data necessary to make a more specific diagnosis are lacking or conflicted. Various descriptive labels have appeared in the clinical literature to identify individuals who show mixed symptom presentations of thought disorders, affective disorders, language disorders, and hyperactivity. Barkley (1990)

Coding Note. Other Specified Schizophrenia Spectrum and Other Psychotic and Brief Psychotic Disorder

Other Specified Schizophrenia Spectrum and Other Psychotic Disorder is the appropriate classification when a case may turn out to meet the criteria for a diagnosis of Brief Psychotic Disorder but the symptoms have not yet remitted (psychotic symptoms have lasted for more than 1 day and less than 1 month, but are still present). If the psychotic symptoms do eventually remit in less than 1 month, the diagnosis should be changed from Other Specified Schizophrenia Spectrum and Other Psychotic Disorder to Brief Psychotic Disorder. (See also the Coding Note on p. 78.)

has discussed children with problems that he calls "multiplex developmental disorders"; Rapoport (1997) has discussed a group of children she refers to as "multidimensionally impaired." In some cases, Other Specified Schizophrenia Spectrum and Other Psychotic Disorder will be resolved into a more specific diagnosis as further information is collected and/or the course of the disorder unfolds. The next Coding Note presents guidelines for distinguishing between Psychotic Disorder Not Otherwise Specified and Brief Psychotic Disorder.

Comorbid and Premorbid Disorders

Epidemiological data suggest that poor childhood adjustment and speech and language disorders may be premorbid risk factors for some of the Psychotic Disorders (Asarnow, 2013). Along with the many other negative prognostic associations for Conduct Disorder is an overrepresentation among adult populations with psychotic diagnoses. Substance Abuse and (less frequently) Substance Dependence are other comorbid problems for individuals with Schizophrenia. The underlying mechanisms driving these associations are unknown and represent a critical area for future investigations.

The three Cluster A Personality Disorders (Schizotypal, Schizoid, Paranoid) have been hypothesized to be associated premorbidly with one or more of the Psychotic Disorders. This hypothesis remains an issue of contention and ongoing interest, but it is certainly of value to attempt to elicit any reliable information possible on premorbid adjustment and personality traits in youth diagnosed with a Psychotic Disorder. The three Cluster A Personality Disorders are made as comorbid diagnoses of Schizophrenia and other Psychotic Disorders only if there is clear evidence that the personality pattern occurs at times other than acute psychotic episodes.

Additional Diagnostic Categories Involving Psychosis

Several Mood Disorders can reach such severity that psychotic symptoms appear. The specifier With Psychotic Features can be used for Major Depressive Episodes that occur in the course of Major Depressive and Bipolar I, as well as for Manic and Mixed Episodes that occur in the course of Bipolar I Disorder.

8

Mood Problems

OVERVIEW

DSM-5 defines *mood* as "a pervasive and sustained emotion that colors the perception of the world" (p. 824). The nature and manifestation of mood problems in youth have received a great deal of attention over recent decades. The idea of serious affective disturbance as a clinical problem in young people, especially children, has been difficult for some investigators to accept, but there has been a growing acknowledgment that mood problems do occur in the young. Furthermore, the accumulated data indicate that although depressive symptoms in children clearly show some developmental features, the overall conceptualizations of depression developed for adults also work for children and adolescents (Cicchetti & Toth, 1998; Kashani, Holcomb, & Orvaschel, 1986; Ryan et al., 1987). Relative to depressive disorders, less is known, and far less is agreed upon, about mania and Bipolar Disorders in children and adolescents (see later discussion), but progress is being made in this area as well (e.g., Birmaher et al., 2014).

When determining diagnosis, the key idea is that the mood disturbance is judged to be the primary feature of the individual's problems. This places a considerable responsibility on the examiner both to be sensitive to indications of depression and other affective disturbances in children and adolescents and to evaluate the complex relations among different symptom clusters and environmental events carefully to arrive at a view of the primary and secondary status of various elements.

Historically, depressive disorders and bipolar disorders (i.e., those that include both symptoms of mania and depression) were included in one DSM chapter covering Mood Disorders. In contrast, DSM-5 separates these kinds of disorders into two chapters, namely "Bipolar and Related Disorders" and "Depressive Disorders." The former chapter is purposely situated in DSM-5 between the chapter covering psychotic disorders (e.g., schizophrenia) and the one covering depressive disorders. This change was intentional: Bipolar disorders were thus sandwiched "in recognition of their place as a bridge between the two diagnostic classes in terms of symptomatology, family history, and genetics" (p. 123). Some research has identified putative common genetic markers and risk factors for Bipolar I Disorder and Schizophrenia.

The chapter on Bipolar and Related Disorders includes seven diagnoses: Bipolar I Disorder, Bipolar II Disorder, Cyclothymic Disorder, Substance/Medication-Induced Bipolar and Related Disorder, Bipolar and Related Disorder Due to Another Medical Condition, Other Specified Bipolar and Related Disorder, and Unspecified Bipolar and Related Disorder. DSM-5 explicitly notes that the Other Specified Bipolar and Related Disorder diagnosis was included to address individuals, including children and adolescents, who display manic and depressive symptomatology but do not meet the full diagnostic criteria for Bipolar I, Bipolar II, or Cyclothymic Disorder.

The chapter on Depressive Disorders includes eight diagnostic categories, including the new diagnosis, Disruptive Mood Dysregulation Disorder, and a long list of specifiers for Depressive Disorders. The diagnoses included in this chapter are: Disruptive Mood Dysregulation Disorder, Major Depressive Disorder, Persistent Depressive Disorder (Dysthymia), Premenstrual Dysphoric Disorder, Substance/Medication-Induced Depressive Disorder, Depressive Disorder Due to Another Medical Condition, Other Specified Depressive Disorder, and Unspecified Depressive Disorder. See the DSM-IV Change Notes later in the chapter for a summary of changes from DSM-IV-TR criteria to the DSM-5 criteria.

These two chapters of DSM-5 bring together most of the syndromes and disorders in this classification system in which mood symptoms are the primary clinical problem. For children and adolescents, the principal additional categories are various forms of Adjustment Disorder involving mood disturbance and Bereavement (covered in DSM-5 in the chapter titled "Conditions for Further Study" in Section III). The IDEA Note on page 86 sets forth how these disorders and conditions relate to eligibility for services under IDEA.

SPECIFIC MOOD DISTURBANCE PATTERNS

DSM-5 focuses on two major mood categories: Mania and Depression. Mania continues to be given primacy as a diagnostic condition: If the criteria for a Manic Episode are present or were ever present, a Bipolar I Disorder diagnosis is indicated. If the criteria of a subthreshold Manic Episode (Hypomania) are met or were ever met, a diagnosis of Bipolar II Disorder is indicated. Current or past episodes of depression with no history of a manic or hypomanic episode may be considered for a Depressive Disorder diagnosis. DSM-5 defines several mood syndromes, which are then used in the criteria for several Mood Disorders. For a detailed discussion of the changes to this diagnostic category from the last edition of DSM, see the DSM-IV Note on page 95. The mood syndromes identified are Manic Episode, Hypomanic Episode, and Major Depressive Episode.

Manic Episode

A Manic Episode is a period of "abnormally and persistently elevated, expansive, or irritable mood and abnormally and persistently increased goal-directed activity or energy" (p. 124). Individuals who experience Manic Episodes tend to feel euphoric, self-confident, grandiose, and irritable; they seem to have endless energy, sleep little, and are busy almost constantly. Poor judgment, excessive pursuit of pleasurable goals, and distractibility may seriously compromise their functional behavior. Psychotic symptoms may also be present during a Manic Episode. A Manic Episode is defined by the presence of the abnormal mood most of the day, nearly every day, for at least 1 week, plus three or more of seven symptoms. Four symptoms are required if the mood is only irritable, as may be more typically the case in children and adolescents. Historically, manic behavior in children was thought to be characterized by irritability and aggressive outbursts and by being more chronic and continuous than in adults (Biederman, 1997), but these ideas have been revisited in recent years and newer ideas about it are reflected in the conceptualization of mania in DSM-5. Specifically, DSM-5 focuses on identifying distinct episodes of manic mood in the diagnosis of Bipolar Disorder. A new diagnosis, Disruptive Mood Dysregulation Disorder, was included in DSM-5 to capture children and adolescents who present with chronic (as opposed to episodic) irritability and angry mood between explosive outbursts. In other words, DSM-5 draws an important distinction between chronic irritability and episodic irritability in terms of differential diagnosis. (See the sections "Disruptive Mood Dysregulation Disorder" and "The Irritable Child," later in this chapter.)

Manic symptoms that are elicited by antidepressant medication, electroconvulsive therapy, light therapy, or other drugs (e.g., corticosteroids) are not considered Manic Episodes and should not be used to document Bipolar I Disorder. If a child with Major Depressive Disorder develops manic behavior in response to treatment with an antidepressant medication, the diagnosis of Major Depressive Disorder remains, and a second diagnosis (Substance-Induced Bipolar and Related Disorder) is added. Such a response to somatic treatment may reflect a bipolar diathesis, and the individual may have an increased likelihood of developing Bipolar I or Bipolar II Disorder in the future. Children and adolescents who show such a response to treatment should be monitored for possible future independent manic symptoms.

Hypomanic Episode

A Hypomanic Episode is a milder form of abnormally elevated mood. The criteria require only 4 days of distinctly different emotional experience characterized by a persistently expansive elevated or irritable mood, plus three of seven additional symptoms (four if the mood disturbance is irritable). Hypomanic Episodes in adolescents may be associated with truancy, delinquent behavior, school failure, or substance use. An episode of hypomanic symptoms in reaction to somatic treatment of depression is not considered a Hypomanic Episode and is not used to establish a diagnosis of Bipolar II Disorder (see the preceding section, "Manic Episode").

Major Depressive Episode

The criteria for a Major Depressive Episode demarcate the boundaries of a serious depressive experience. Five of nine defining symptoms are required to be in evidence for a minimum of 2 weeks. These symptoms represent a change from the individual's previous level of functioning and cause either significant distress or functional impairment. One of the five or more symptoms used to document a Major Depressive Episode in a child or adolescent must be either (1) depressed or irritable mood (in adults, only depressed mood is considered) or (2) loss of interest or pleasure. One of the remaining symptoms is also modified for children: Rather than the adult criterion of weight loss, the failure to show expected developmental weight gain can be considered a symptom of depression in children. There is discussion in the text of other developmental features of depression in youth. Somatic complaints, agitation and restlessness, and mood-congruent hallucinations may be more frequent in depression in prepubescent children. Adolescents may be more likely to show acting-out and conduct problems, substance misuse, and declining academic performance and achievement. Symptoms of mania preclude identification of a Major Depressive Episode, but symptoms of psychosis do not.

IDEA Note. Mood-Related Disorders/Conditions and IDEA

A DSM-5 diagnosis of a mental disorder or condition centering around mood can be used to support qualifying a child for special education services under the "serious emotional disturbance" category of IDEA. A "general pervasive mood of unhappiness or depression" that persists "over a period of time" and "adversely affects educational performance" is one of the defining conditions indicating a "serious emotional disturbance" (Individuals with Disabilities Education Improvement Act [IDEA], 2004, Public Law 108-446, paragraph (c)(4)(i)). Another identified condition is "an inability to build or maintain satisfactory relationships with peers and teachers," which is a common symptom of Depressive or Bipolar Disorders in children and adolescents. Documentation of the functional impairment in academic or social adjustment caused by the mood disturbance is important. Beyond the diagnosis, additional psychosocial and environmental characteristics of the child and evaluation of the child's functioning may also be important in establishing eligibility for services under IDEA.

The IDEA description of severe emotional disturbance has been criticized on several grounds, including the requirement that the qualifying condition must have a negative influence on educational performance. It is certainly possible that a bright child could maintain adequate scholastic performance even under the burden of severe depression, for example, but typically depression will cause a decline in the quality of schoolwork. An unexplained deterioration in school performance is often an early overt symptom of Major Depressive Disorder in children and adolescents. Clarizio and Payette's (1990) survey of school psychologists' practice with respect to childhood depression suggested a much greater reliance on the operational criteria of the DSM than on Public Law 94-142. This practice probably continues to be the case with DSM-5 and IDEA.

MENTAL DISORDERS INVOLVING MOOD

Bipolar I Disorder, Bipolar II Disorder, Cyclothymic Disorder, and Other Specified and Unspecified Bipolar Disorder

Manic Episodes are rare in children (<1% of cases; Biederman, 1997; Emslie, Kennard, & Kowatch, 1995) and not common in adolescents. However, they do occur, and they are probably often missed because of evaluators' failure to consider them possibilities. Bipolar I Disorder involves a current episode or past history of at least one full-blown Manic Episode meeting the DSM-5 diagnostic criteria; there may or may not be a history of Major Depressive Episodes. Bipolar II Disorder involves a current episode or past history of at least one Major Depressive and at least one Hypomanic Episode (mild manic syndrome). Cyclothymic Disorder in children and adolescents involves at least 1 year of "numerous periods with hypomanic symptoms" and "numerous periods with depressive symptoms" that never meet full criteria for a Manic Episode or a Major Depressive Episode. Other Specified Bipolar and Related Disorder and Unspecified Bipolar and Related Disorder cover a number of possible combinations of mood symptoms that do not meet the criteria for any specific Bipolar Disorder.

Differential Diagnosis

Carlson and Meyer (2006), Emslie and colleagues (1995), and Geller and Luby (1997) discuss reasons why Bipolar Disorders are difficult to diagnose in childhood and adolescence and give examples of behavior in children that reflect the DSM criteria for these disorders. Earlier, Weinberg and Brumback (1976) presented alternative criteria for mania in children. A review of this material may be helpful in sensitizing an examiner to possible signs of manic behavior, but a formal diagnosis of Bipolar Disorder requires the documentation of symptoms that meet the DSM-5 criteria.

In older clients, confidence in correctly determining differential diagnosis of Bipolar Disorders and Attention-Deficit/Hyperactivity Disorder increases (Carr, 2009). Bipolar Disorders in adolescents are expected to be episodic and relatively uninfluenced by environmental settings and contingencies; Attention-Deficit/Hyperactivity Disorder, in contrast, tends to be a consistent problem but does clearly vary in response to situation and feedback. The situation is complicated by evidence that Attention-Deficit/Hyperactivity Disorder and Bipolar Disorders may be associated (Biederman, 1997). There have been cases reported that initially presented as Attention-Deficit/Hyperactivity Disorder and that later appeared to develop into a Bipolar Disorder (Yaylayan, Tumuluru, Weller, & Weller, 1996). Birmaher and colleagues (1996) report that greater attention to the possibility of Bipolar II Disorder in adolescents is important because the symptoms of this Mood Disorder can easily be mistaken for those of a Disruptive Behavior Disorder or a Personality Disorder, especially Borderline Personality Disorder. Geller and Luby (1997), in the review discussed previously, argue that Bipolar Disorders are underdiagnosed in children because of age-specific developmental features in presentation and course.

The differentiation of Bipolar Disorders from Schizophrenia in adolescents (and possibly children) can be problematic as well. Adolescent-onset mania may present more often with psychotic symptoms that are misdiagnosed as Schizophrenia (McGlashan, 1988). Werry (1996, p. 33) has suggested that the following features are more common in child and adolescent psychosis due to Bipolar Disorders (as opposed to Schizophrenia): (1) lack of developmental abnormalities, (2) acute (rapid) onset, and (3) a family history of Bipolar Disorders. Geller and Luby (1997) also stress a family history of mania as an important aid in differentiating Bipolar Disorders from Schizophrenia in adolescents.

Other possibilities to be considered in the differential diagnosis of Bipolar Disorders in teenagers are the Substance-Related Disorders. Both can lead to abrupt changes in usual behavior, emotional symptoms, and deteriorating adjustment and school performance. This challenge is further complicated by the possibility that Bipolar Disorders in youth may occur more characteristically with rapid cycling and hence may be less distinct from the "highs" and "lows" produced by substance use. Moreover, there is high comorbidity between actual Bipolar Disorder and Substance-Related Disorders; in particular, many adolescents with Bipolar I Disorder will begin or increase substance use, along with the other behavior excesses of a Manic Episode. A careful review of a young person's substance use history, with multiple informants if possible, is strongly advised in any evaluation for possible Bipolar Disorders in youth.

Geller and Luby (1997) recommend that young people being evaluated for possible Bipolar Disorders also be evaluated for possible Communication Disorders. A young person may present with disorganized speech that suggests a thought disorder, but this symptom may actually reflect a primary language disturbance. The youth's need to communicate and frantic attempts to do so may be interpreted as a flight of ideas or pressured speech. Youth with manic symptoms are highly distractible and can show looseness of associations, but they do not have any fundamental language problem.

Another consideration for differential diagnosis of Bipolar Disorders involves a presentation of hypersexual behavior. Excessive goal-directed activity is a cardinal symptom of mania, and one common manifestation is an increase in sexual speech, sexual behavior, and sexual acting out. Uncharacteristic profanity, poorly concealed masturbation, ill-considered propositioning of potential sexual partners, romantic fantasies with delusional qualities, use of telephone or online sex services (e.g., "1-900" calls), and dangerous sexual behavior (e.g., unprotected sex, multiple partners, little or no discrimination in selection of sexual partners) may all be symptomatic of a Manic Episode in older children and adolescents. These behaviors may also reflect a history of sexual abuse, and a careful evaluation of this possibility is called for whenever the school psychologist is confronted with unusual sexual activity in a young person.

In female adolescents a final differential to consider is Premenstrual Dysphoric Disorder. Although a certain amount of controversy has surrounded this category, it seems undeniable that a small percentage of post-pubertal women experience luteal phase mood swings of sufficient severity to cause significant personal distress, if not impairments in interpersonal functioning. This occurrence may be underrecognized in clinical populations because of continuing social and personal sensitivity and stigma associated with menstruation. However, charting of daily mood ratings for most women suffering from depressive or bipolar disorders will show little or no covariation with their menstrual cycle, and the differential diagnosis can usually be arrived at with confidence.

Heuristic for Suspecting Mania in Children and Adolescents

A positive family history of Bipolar Disorders is strongly associated with manic-depressive behavior (Carr, 2009; Isaac, 1991), and Bipolar Disorders should be included among the diagnostic considerations in any child or adolescent with such a family history. In addition, we recommend a consideration of Bipolar Disorders in children exhibiting disruptive behavior who are also reported to have exhibited the following characteristics:

1. Irritable moods lasting for sustained periods (days to weeks).
2. Labile, unstable moods (mood changes in response to minimal provocation).
3. Incidents of explosive aggression that are poorly organized and seem nonfunctional.
4. Poor response to usually effective treatments.
5. A history of Attention-Deficit/Hyperactivity Disorder diagnosis with fluctuating symptoms or responses to treatment.

One difficulty in evaluating children or adolescents suspected of having a possible Bipolar Disorder is determining family history of mental disorders. DMS-5 notes that a family history of Bipolar Disorder "is one of the strongest and most consistent risk factors for bipolar disorder" (p. 130). Many other researchers (e.g., Carr, 2009; Isaac, 1991) identify family history as a significant risk factor for manic and hypomanic syndromes and bipolar disorders. The question is: How confident are we in the family history offered by the parents or other collaterals interviewed? It is one thing to have a family history that includes one or more individuals formally diagnosed with a Bipolar Disorder by a mental health professional after a comprehensive evaluation; another thing to have a diagnosis of Bipolar Disorder listed on a medical record based only on the client's self-report; and another to have a parent proclaim that his or her child "must be bipolar because he [she] snaps out." These are all relevant data to consider, but differential weights would probably be assigned to each. In the recent past a label of "depression" was often given by family members to individuals

DSM-IV Note. Changes in DSM-5 for Bipolar and Related Disorders

Both Bipolar Disorders and Depressive Disorders were housed in one chapter, "Mood Disorders" in DSM-IV-TR. These disorder categories are each given their own chapters in DSM-5, namely "Bipolar and Related Disorders" and "Depressive Disorders." Bipolar Disorders are presented first, demonstrating the primacy of the presence of a manic or subthreshold manic episode in determining diagnosis. That is, manic or hypomanic symptoms are associated with diagnoses within the Bipolar category (e.g., Bipolar I, Bipolar II, Cyclothymic Disorder, Substance/Medication-Induced Bipolar and Related Disorder). DSM-5 also discontinued Mixed Episodes as a distinct category and added it to the extensive list of specifiers for Bipolar Disorders. It is worth noting that these specifiers also include Bipolar Disorders induced by medical conditions, medication, and other substances, which were formerly given their own diagnostic criteria in DSM-IV-TR. Specific changes to the DSM criteria for Bipolar and Related Disorders are detailed below.

Bipolar I Disorder

DSM-IV-TR provides separate diagnostic criteria for six different presentations of Bipolar I Disorder based on the primary characteristics of the most recent episode (e.g., Single Manic Episode, Most Recent Episode Depressed). DSM-5 includes all of these presentations as one disorder, Bipolar I Disorder, with different ICD codes for the various presentations provided in tables. In contrast with DSM-IV-TR, Criterion A for Manic and Hypomanic Episodes in DSM-5 now includes the statement that symptoms must be "present most of the day, nearly every day" (p. 124). Similarly, Criterion B now requires that the symptoms represent a "change from usual behavior" (p. 124).

Bipolar II Disorder

No major changes were made to the diagnostic criteria for this disorder.

Cyclothymic Disorder

DSM-5 requires that the depressive or hypomanic episodes must be present for at least half the time during a 1-year period of symptoms. DSM-5 also requires that the criteria for a major mood disorder (i.e., Major Depressive Disorder, Bipolar I, Bipolar II) have never been met. If the criteria for one of these disorders are met, the individual is no longer eligible for a Cyclothymic Disorder diagnosis. DSM-5 added a new specifier, With Anxious Distress, to the list of specifiers for this and the other bipolar disorders.

hospitalized for serious psychiatric disorders, some of whom probably had a Depressive Disorder, whereas others had a Bipolar Disorder and still others had Schizophrenia or another Psychotic Disorder. Currently, "being bipolar" seems to have become the acceptable expression for any recurrent lapse of behavior or impulse control. Although some of these individuals probably are "Bipolar" in the DSM-5 sense of the term, many are not. This common mislabeling is not, of course, an issue restricted to Bipolar Disorder. Our conclusions can be no better than the data on which these conclusions are based. The information provided by parents, teachers, and other informants can be invaluable in arriving at the clearest understanding of a youth's situation, as long as we remember that these are communications from another person and subject to all the possible influences that implies.

Disruptive Mood Dysregulation Disorder

One of the most interesting changes to DSM-5 is the inclusion of a new category within the Depressive Disorders chapter, Disruptive Mood Dysregulation Disorder. It is the stated intent of DSM-5 to address some of the many concerns that have been raised regarding the possible overdiagnosis of Bipolar Disorder in youth, especially the overdiagnosis of the previous DSM-IV-TR category of Bipolar Disorder Not Otherwise Specified. Another related concern may have been the greatly increased off-label use of neuroleptic medications for treatment of children and adolescents with these diagnoses. Whether adding this new category will address adequately either of these two issues will have to be seen.

The inclusion of the diagnosis in the "Depressive Disorder" chapter, as opposed to the "Bipolar" chapter or the "Disruptive Behavior Disorders" chapter, is a further interesting issue. The chapter introduction suggests that this placement is justified by evidence that these youth tend to have unipolar depressive or anxiety disorders upon follow-up as adults. It does seem to be the case that the majority of these individuals do not go on to develop classic Bipolar diagnoses. The issue of where and how to draw diagnostic boundaries is one of the major challenges in developing the most useful categorical systems. All of this aside, practitioners of child psychology, psychiatry, and allied disciplines have a new diagnostic category with which to contend. The full influence of this new classification will have to be evaluated over the coming years.

The category of Disruptive Mood Dysregulation Disorder is conceptualized as a pattern of "persistent irritability and frequent episodes of extreme behavioral dyscontrol" (p. 155) as manifested in severe and recurrent temper outbursts with persistent irritable or angry mood predominating in between outbursts, with an onset before age 10. The diagnosis should not be given prior to age 6. There seems to be some disagreement within the text as to what age span this diagnosis is appropriate for after the age of 6. The introduction to the chapter mentions "up to 12 years of age" (p. 155); the diagnostic criteria indicates the diagnosis should not be made for the first time "after age 18" (p. 156); the Development and Course section suggests that "use of the diagnosis should be restricted to age groups similar to those in which validity has been established (7–18 years)." It appears the intent was to restrict use of this diagnosis to a span of 6 to 18 years.

Great attention is paid to differentiating as clearly as possible between Disruptive Mood Dysregulation Disorder and Bipolar Disorders. The practitioner should carefully consider the Diagnostic Criteria, Diagnostic Features, and the Differential Diagnosis sections when considering use of this diagnosis. The diagnosis of Disruptive Mood Dysregulation Disorder cannot be given currently with one of Oppositional Defiant Disorder, Intermittent Explosive Disorder, or Bipolar Disorder; it can be made concurrently with Major Depressive Disorder, Attention-Deficit/Hyperactivity Disorder, Conduct Disorder, and Substance Use Disorder. The text does give one explicit decision rule: If the child meets criteria for both Disruptive Mood Dysregulation Disorder and Oppositional Defiant Disorder, only the Disruptive Mood Dysregulation Disorder diagnosis is given.

Major Depressive Disorder

Major Depressive Disorder (known as Major Depressive Disorder in DSM-IV and DSM-IV-TR, but listed as Major Depression in DSM-III and DSM-III-R) is diagnosed on the basis of full manifestation of a Major Depressive Episode (five of nine criteria are required, as noted earlier) for 2 weeks or more in a child or adolescent. One of the (minimum) five symptoms must be either sustained dysphoric mood or anhedonia. In children, irritability, as well as sadness, is considered a dysphoric mood.

For a child, we recommend a differential consideration of possible Major Depressive Disorder if the examiner is confronted with repeated somatic complaints without apparent explanation, a perception by others (teacher, parents, peers) that the child is unhappy or seems sad, or an unexplained deterioration in school performance or behavior. The index of sensitivity is markedly increased in cases in which there is a family history of a mood disorder. Anxiety is a frequently associated symptom of depression in children and adolescents (Cummings, Caporino, & Kendall, 2014; Garber & Weersing, 2010; Tumuluru, Yaylayan, Weller, & Weller, 1996). Any prior history of serious depression is a significant risk factor for subsequent clinical depressions. Major Depressive Disorder is specified as Single Episode or Recurrent. Whereas the Single Episode type is a risk factor for future depression, the Recurrent type almost guarantees recurrence of Major Depressive Episodes over the lifespan and justifies appropriate planning.

A specifier available in DSM-5 for Major Depressive Disorder is With Seasonal Pattern. More commonly referred to as "seasonal affective disorder," the occurrence of some severe depressions at particular times of the year (usually fall or winter) is now well accepted. Often associated with excessive sleeping, overeating, craving for carbohydrate-rich foods, and weight gain, seasonal affective disorder has gained increasing attention in investigations of recurrent depressions in adults but little systematic study in children (Giedd, Swedo, Lowe, & Rosenthal, 1998). Despite the limited empirical literature, there is good reason to conclude that seasonal affective disorder does occur in children and is often missed in evaluations. Giedd and colleagues (1998) present a series of case studies of youngsters followed over 7 years with diagnoses of seasonal affective disorder. They suggest that a pattern of best school performance in the first and last quarters, with deterioration of academic achievement in the second and third quarters, may indicate the presence of this disorder. Their literature review suggests a 3% estimated prevalence of seasonal affective disorder in children; the majority of these cases are not diagnosed. Sensitivity to this diagnostic possibility could be a valuable service of the school psychologist.

Persistent Depressive Disorder (Dysthymia)

Persistent Depressive Disorder (Dysthymia or Depressive Neurosis in DSM-III, DSM-III-R, DSM-IV, and DSM-IV-TR) identifies a chronic depressive state of less severity than the more florid Major Depressive Disorder. As with Major Depressive Disorder, important developmental modifications for Persistent Depressive Disorder in children and adolescents have been made in both the defining mood criteria and the duration criteria. The negative mood, as in Major Depressive Disorder, can be one of either depression or irritability (depressed mood is required in adults); in addition, the duration required for diagnosis is reduced from 2 years (for adults) to 1 year. During the period of negative mood, two out of six additional symptoms are required. Kashani, Allan, Beck, Bledsoe, and Reid (1997) discuss the relative usefulness of different informants (child, parent, teacher) in gathering data on dysthymic symptoms in young children. Especially in younger children, the presentation of Persistent Depressive Disorder may differ from the typical clinical picture. Kashani's group found psychomotor agitation, aggressive behavior, and somatic complaints (none of which are DSM-5 symptoms of Persistent Depressive Disorder) to be common in a group of preschool children diagnosed with this disorder (75%, 100%, and 100%, respectively; Kashani et al., 1997, p. 1431).

During the 1-year duration of Persistent Depressive Disorder required in children and adolescents, it is specified that the young person must never have been free from symptoms for a period of 2 months or more. The development of a full-blown Major Depressive Episode at any time during the initial year of Persistent Depressive Disorder preempts the diagnosis of Persistent Depressive Disorder, and the youth is diagnosed with Major Depressive Disorder instead. After the 1-year "qualifying period" for Persistent Depressive Disorder, a Major Depressive Episode superimposed on Persistent Depressive Disorder receives a second diagnosis (Persistent Depressive Disorder and Major Depressive Disorder); in much of the psychological literature, this situation is referred to as "dual depression." Appearance of a Manic Episode or Hypomanic Episode preempts the diagnosis of Persistent Depressive Disorder, and the diagnosis of either Bipolar I or Bipolar II Disorder is given instead; any history of Cyclothymic Disorder preempts the diagnosis of Persistent Depressive Disorder.

Substance/Medication-Induced Disorders

In children and adolescents, a disturbance in mood can develop as a consequence of substance use (Substance/Medication-Induced Bipolar and Related Disorder and Substance/Medication-Induced Depressive Disorder) or of a general medical condition (Bipolar and Related Disorder Due to Another Medical Condition and Depressive Disorder Due to Another Medical Condition). That is, symptoms of depression, mania, or both may develop during drug or medication intoxication or withdrawal, as well as in response to illness, injury, or some other physiological influence.

Other Specified and Unspecified Disorders

Other Specified Bipolar and Related Disorder and Unspecified Bipolar and Related Disorder are residual categories for clinical pictures that (1) meet the general criteria for one of these categories of mental disorder and (2) do not meet the criteria for any specific Bipolar Disorder. Similar categories are offered for depressive mood: Other Specified Depressive Disorder and Unspecified Depressive Disorder. These diagnoses are not made concurrently with another specific mood disorder. The presence of atypical features or symptoms may be noted after a specific mood disorder, but these should not be classified as a separate additional diagnosis. The categories can be diagnosed in association with other general groups of diagnoses if the key symptoms (i.e., manic or depressive symptoms) are not common associated symptoms of that disorder. For instance, Other Specified Depressive Disorder may be diagnosed in association with Obsessive–Compulsive Disorder, but it should not be diagnosed concurrently with Schizophrenia

DSM-IV Note. Changes in DSM-5 for Depressive Disorders

Beyond the separation of Depressive Disorders from Bipolar Disorders in one chapter on "Mood Disorders," the biggest change to the Depressive Disorders section of the DSM is the addition of a new diagnostic category, Disruptive Mood Dysregulation Disorder. This new disorder is discussed elsewhere in this chapter and in "The Irritable Child" section in this chapter. Other specific changes to the depressive disorders most relevant to the schools are detailed here. As with other chapters, the DSM replaced the Not Otherwise Specified category with Other Specified and Unspecified categories in the fifth edition. DSM-5 also includes an extensive list of specifiers for Depressive Disorders. It is worth noting that these specifiers include Depressive Disorders induced by medical conditions, medication, and other substances, which were formerly given their own diagnostic criteria in DSM-IV-TR.

Major Depressive Disorder

The diagnostic criteria now provide more explicit leeway for the clinician to give the diagnosis of Major Depressive Disorder concurrent with bereavement.

Persistent Depressive Disorder (Dysthymia)

Other than a name change (i.e., Dysthymic Disorder to Persistent Depressive Disorder), the criteria are largely the same. The list of specifiers is more extensive. In DSM-IV-TR, specifiers were provided for onset and atypical features. In DSM-5, the list of specifiers has expanded to include not only onset (i.e., Early vs. Late) and atypical features, but a whole host of other features (i.e., With Anxious Distress, With Mixed Features, With Melancholic Features, With Atypical Features, With Mood-Congruent Psychotic Features, With Mood-Incongruent Psychotic Features, and With Peripartum Onset), as well as remission status (i.e., In Partial Remission or In Full Remission), severity (i.e., Mild, Moderate, or Severe), and involvement of other mood disorders (i.e., With Pure Dysthymic Syndrome, With Persistent Major Depressive Episode, With Intermittent Major Depressive Episode, With Current Episode, With Intermittent Major Depressive Episode, Without Current Episode).

Premenstrual Dysphoric Disorder

Formerly included as a criteria set in need of further study in DSM-IV-TR, Premenstrual Dysphoric Disorder is included as a Mental Disorder in the "Depressive Disorders" chapter of DSM-5. The criteria are basically the same in the two editions of the DSM, although there are a few differences. DSM-5 includes the requirement that the problems are not better accounted for by a medical condition or a substance (e.g., medication, other treatment). DSM-5 uses less medical jargon in describing the timing of symptoms than did its predecessor. That is, DSM-5 describes the symptoms relative to the weeks leading up to and following onset of menses, whereas DSM-IV-TR detailed the symptoms in terms of menstrual phase (e.g., luteal, follicular phase); thus DSM-5 makes the language more accessible to nonphysicians.

because depressive symptoms are commonly associated features of this Psychotic Disorder.

OTHER MOOD-RELATED DISORDERS AND CONDITIONS

Adjustment Disorders Involving Mood Disturbance

As noted previously, an Adjustment Disorder is a Mental Disorder; that is, it must fall within the general parameters of a Mental Disorder as defined by DSM-5 (clinically significant distress, impairment of adaptive behavior, or specific outcome risks). Adjustment Disorders in general are defined by the development of clinically significant symptoms in response to an identified psychosocial stress or stressors. Adjustment Disorders are excluded if the symptoms meet the criteria for an alternative, specific disorder, even if a known stressor precipitates this disorder. Adjustment Disorders in DSM-5 are classifications of exclusion; only if no other diagnosable pattern accounts for the symptoms seen is an Adjustment Disorder diagnosis allowed. Adjustment Disorders can be diagnosed concurrently with other diagnoses, but only when novel problems have developed that are not associated with the previously diagnosed Mental Disorders and when these symptoms have a clear precipitating event.

Adjustment Disorder is subtyped by the predominant symptoms experienced. Three of the five specific subtypes are relevant to this section: Adjustment Disorder With Depressed Mood, Adjustment Disorder With Mixed Anxiety and Depressed Mood, and Adjustment Disorder With Mixed Disturbance of Emotions (depression, anxiety) and Conduct. There is also an Unspecified subtype to cover other behavioral reactions. The diagnosis of Adjustment Disorder is usually not made if the symptom picture of depression occurs in response to a death; rather, the diagnosis of Bereavement is given.

Bereavement

One of several controversies that emerged as preliminary versions of DSM-5 were presented for review and comment by different clinicians, investigators, and professional bodies was the removal of the Bereavement exclusion from Major Depressive Disorder. In DSM-IV, the condition of Bereavement (not a Mental Disorder in DSM-IV but an Additional Condition That May Be a Focus of Clinical Attention) precluded a diagnosis of Major Depressive Disorder for approximately 2 months. DSM-5 removes this precluding relation between loss of a loved one and serious depression and gives the clinician the opportunity and task of differentiating between normal grief, which can be incredibly intense and disruptive, and clinical depression, a mental disorder. DSM-5 also includes, in the chapter on "Conditions for Further Study," proposed criteria and discussion for a possible Persistent Complex Bereavement Disorder diagnosis. (This diagnosis would not be made in DSM-5 as it is currently written.)

Persistent Complex Bereavement Disorder is provided in DSM-5 as a proposed criteria set for research purposes (i.e., it is not a mental disorder as defined in DSM-5 but is included as a Condition for Further Study). The criteria for Persistent Complex Bereavement Disorder clearly differentiate between normal and psychopathological grief reactions. This discussion emphasizes symptoms that are not typically seen in normal grief. It is somewhat similar to the "complicated grief disorder" proposed by Horowitz and colleagues (1997). The description includes a specifier, With Traumatic Bereavement, for cases of traumatic loss through homicide or suicide. In general, the differential diagnosis of Major Depressive Disorder and Bereavement requires consideration of the symptoms presented; the survivor's expressed distress and personal interpretation of the symptoms experienced; the functional status of the survivor with respect to his or her major obligations (school, family responsibilities, social relationships); the survivor's cultural and family background; the survivor's relationship with the deceased; and the duration and course of the survivor's reaction to the death.

Loss of a loved one is a challenging topic upon which to attempt to formulate distinct categories with general applicability. Cultures, subcultures, societies, communities, families, and individuals vary incredibly in their beliefs and thoughts about death and how to respond appropriately to this shared human reality. The best guidance we can offer on this topic is to proceed cautiously and with great humility.

The Irritable Child

More than any previous edition of DSM, the fifth edition has incorporated greater guidance in classifying children and adolescents who present with irritability. This change is likely in response to a stated growing concern about the overdiagnosis of Bipolar Disorder in children that does not follow the same developmental presentation as that found in adults. That is, children diagnosed with Bipolar Disorder are more likely to have diagnoses of Depressive and/or Anxiety Disorders in adulthood than they are to maintain a Bipolar Disorder diagnosis (p. 155). Consistent with this observation, Leibenluft, Cohen, Gorrindo, Brook, and Pine (2006) found differences in sequelae for episodic presentations of irritability relative to chronic presentations. Specifically, they found a pattern of early adulthood diagnosis of mania in children who initially presented with episodic irritability, whereas children who presented initially with chronic irritability were more likely to have the diagnosis of depression in early adulthood. These findings highlight the importance of a thorough assessment of the duration and character of irritability. In addition, evaluating its medical, behavioral, and situational concomitants is crucial for accurate diagnosis and treatment (First, 2014).

Irritable mood or irritability in children appears in the diagnostic criteria for several disorders, including:

Bipolar and Related Disorders
- Bipolar I Disorder
- Bipolar II Disorder
- Cyclothymic Disorder
- Substance/Medication-Induced Bipolar and Related Disorder
- Bipolar and Related Disorder Due to Another Medical Condition
- Other Specified Bipolar and Related Disorder
- Unspecified Bipolar and Related Disorder

Depressive Disorders
- Disruptive Mood Dysregulation Disorder
- Major Depressive Disorder
- Persistent Depressive Disorder
- Premenstrual Dysphoric Disorder
- Substance/Medication-Induced Depressive Disorder
- Depressive Disorder Due to Another Medical Condition
- Other Specified Depressive Disorder
- Unspecified Depressive Disorder

Disruptive, Impulse-Control, and Conduct Disorder
- Oppositional Defiant Disorder

Personality Disorders
- Antisocial Personality Disorder
- Borderline Personality Disorder

Trauma- or Stress-Related Disorders
- Posttraumatic Stress Disorder
- Acute Stress Disorder
- Adjustment Disorder Unspecified

Fortunately, DSM-5 provides guidance for differential diagnosis among these disorders. In the *DSM-5 Handbook of Differential Diagnosis*, First (2014) also spells out nicely many of the considerations regarding irritable mood in a detailed decision tree. This author provides direction for some clinical decision making related to the irritable child; however, First does not include coverage of irritability in reaction to a specific stressor, as we do here.

Generally, decision making begins with a rule-out of a medical explanation for the irritability, including use of a substance or its withdrawal as an explanation for the irritability. If no medical explanation is found, then careful examination of its duration is in order. Does the child present with distinct episodes of irritability? If so, is the irritability coupled with increased activity, or is it seen with other signs of depression? In the former, a Bipolar and Related Disorder diagnosis may be appropriate. In the latter, a Depressive Disorder diagnosis may be appropriate. If the irritability is chronic, as opposed to episodic, a diagnosis of Disruptive Mood Dysregulation Disorder or Oppositional Defiant Disorder may be warranted. If the irritability is chronic and coupled with extreme emotional outbursts, and the child is between 6 and 18 years old with onset of symptoms before 10 years old, the new diagnosis of Disruptive Mood Dysregulation Disorder may be most appropriate. (Disruptive Mood Dysregulation Disorder is contrasted with Intermittent Explosive Disorder, which lacks the chronic irritability seen in Disruptive Mood Dysregulation Disorder and captures individuals who present with repeated, extreme, aggressive outbursts.) If, however, the chronic irritability is coupled with anger, vindictiveness, and disobedience, a diagnosis of Oppositional Defiant Disorder may be warranted. In cases in which the irritability appears to be characterological, a Personality Disorder diagnosis in adults, but not in children, may be appropriate. Finally, if the irritability is in response to or following an identifiable, distressing event, a diagnosis of one of the Trauma- or Stress-Related Disorders, such as Posttraumatic Stress Disorder, Acute Stress Disorder, or Adjustment Disorder Unspecified, may be appropriate.

It is probably worth noting here that there is little empirical evidence to support this process of decision making and the current distinctions between some of these disorders. For example, Burke and colleagues (2014) present results that call into question the distinction between Oppositional Defiant Disorder and the new Disruptive Mood Dysregulation Disorder. With the DSM-5 and its new diagnostic categories in their infancy, it is impossible to know how readily the changes will be adopted and how well they will match the patterns of symptoms shown in clinical settings. Only time will tell.

In the meantime, it is worth considering what the implications of this information might be on practice in the schools. The short answer is that it could make a big difference in terms of eligibility for special education services for a child who presents with irritability. All of the disorders discussed in relation to irritability have an underlying emotional component. Therefore, the presence of one or more of these disorders could readily provide the documentation that would qualify a child for special education services if this emotional disturbance is adversely affecting his or her school performance.

Importantly, this change in conceptualization of irritability as an emotional disturbance in DSM-5 could lead to increases in the number of children who did not qualify for special education services in the past but may now be considered. For example, a child diagnosed with both Conduct Disorder and Oppositional Defiant Disorder, a combination that was previously forbidden in DSM-IV-TR, might be deemed eligible for special education services because of the emotional disturbance underlying the Oppositional Defiant Disorder. Previously, this child may have been labeled "socially maladjusted" with the singular diagnosis of Conduct Disorder and excluded from services under IDEA. Thus, these changes could have major implications for the number of children served.

ISSUES IN THE EVALUATION OF MOOD DISORDERS

The initial concern about children and adolescents with mood disorders will often be precipitated by a change in the young person's level of performance or adjustment. Indeed, DSM-5 emphasizes observation of a noted change in functioning when applying the diagnostic criteria for mood disorders to children. In particular, school psychologists mention motivational changes as a primary expression of depression in school settings (Clarizio & Payette, 1990). Deterioration in quality of academic performance, withdrawal from social and extracurricular activities, and/or the appearance of behavior problems in the absence of any history of acting out are examples of the negative changes in youth that both prompt caretaker concern and raise a question of possible mood disturbance. Although Mood Disorders in children may be less episodic than in adults, a recent change in a child's adjustment is an important cue. Even with more enduring presentations (e.g., Dysthymic Disorder), helping professionals are often rewarded for asking this question: "Has the child always been like this?"

Developmental Trends

Although there is evidence of significant correlations between various mood disorders, these patterns can be supported as distinct clinical phenomena in children (Cicchetti & Toth, 1998; Keller, 1994; Simeon, 1989). An awareness of developmental trends is valuable, especially in school settings, where a child may be followed over years. Persistent Depressive Disorder often shows the earliest age of onset among the mood disorders and can be identified in some children as early as preschool (Kashani et al., 1997). Some cases of Persistent Depressive Disorder follow a continuous or intermittent course throughout an individual's life, whereas others evolve into other mood disorder patterns. The earlier the onset of the Persistent Depressive Disorder, the greater the likelihood of other comorbid disorders. In approximately 70% of cases of early-onset Persistent Depressive Disorder, the young person will eventually develop Major Depressive Disorder (Birmaher et al., 1996). Major Depressive Disorder tends to be episodic; Persistent Depressive Disorder may or may not be evident during periods of recovery from the Major Depressive Disorder. Finally, between 20 and 40% of adolescents with a diagnosis of Major Depressive Disorder will develop Bipolar I Disorder within 5 years (Birmaher et al., 1996).

Developmental trends are also evident in the emerging literature on Bipolar Disorders in children and adolescents. As just noted, a number of adolescents with an initial presentation of depression will eventually "switch" to a manic symptom picture. In adolescents, the manic presentation is often an adult-pattern onset—abrupt, discontinuous with previous adjustment, responsive to treatment, and fully resolved between episodes (Geller & Luby, 1997). There is some evidence that the presentation of episodic irritability, in contrast with chronic irritability, shows continuity in the expression of Bipolar Disorder in early adulthood (Leibenluft et al., 2009). As mentioned previously, presentation in children has been a controversial topic that has been addressed by DSM-5 in part with the addition of a new diagnosis, Disruptive Mood Dysregulation Disorder.

Comorbidity

Comorbidity is the rule rather than the exception for mood disorders as defined by DSM-5, complicating the task for the examiner. Birmaher and colleagues' (1996) review reported that among youth with Major Depressive Disorder, 40–70% have another psychiatric diagnosis, with 20–50% having two or more comorbid diagnoses. The most frequently reported comorbid disorders with Major Depressive Disorder are Persistent Depressive Disorder, Anxiety Disorders, Attention-Deficit/Hyperactivity Disorder and other Disruptive Behavior Disorders, and Substance-Related Disorder. In a more recent study of 201 children and 715 adolescents with Major Depressive Disorder, Yorbik, Birmaher, Axelson, Williamson, and Ryan (2004) found a comorbid Anxiety Disorder in nearly 35% of children and 28% of adolescents, comorbid Attention-Deficit/Hyperactivity Disorder in 15% of children and 6% of adolescents, a comorbid Disruptive Behavior Disorder in 23% of children and 19% of adolescents, and substance abuse in 1% of children and 11% of adolescents. Especially for other internalizing disorders, it may be difficult to establish a clear case for asserting an independent diagnosis, as opposed to considering the other internalizing symptoms as associated symptoms of the Major Depressive Disorder, particularly in light of recent research linking anxiety and depression in youth (Cummings et al., 2014). The methodological difficulties associated with evaluating emotional problems relative to conduct disturbances in children are another major stumbling block here, and often only repeated assessments involving multiple informants can clarify the clinical picture. The overall directive is relatively clear: Isolated symptoms of anxiety can be considered associated symptoms of Major Depressive Disorder; an Anxiety Disorder, however, should be recognized if it is occurring and diagnosed if it meets full criteria.

Reviews of Bipolar Disorders in children and adolescents (Carlson & Meyer, 2006; Geller & Luby, 1997) noted similar high frequencies of comorbidity with other behavior problems. Among children seen for evaluation of Bipolar Disorders, almost 90% have a history of Attention-Deficit/Hyperactivity Disorder; among adolescents, the prevalence is 30% (Geller et al., 1995). Conduct Disorder has been diagnosed in approximately 22% of children and 18% of adolescents evaluated with a Bipolar Disorder (Geller et al., 1995). Carlson and Meyer (2006) report that instances of noncomorbidity range from low to nonexistent, reflecting that comorbidity with Bipolar is the rule rather than the exception. These results raise conceptual questions: Do Attention-Deficit/Hyperactivity Disorder and the Disruptive Behavior Disorders seen in youth prior to a diagnosis of a Bipolar Disorder constitute the initial presentation of the mood disorder, or are they separate comorbid conditions? The high reported comorbidities also present challenges for differential diagnosis. Anxiety Disorders are common in children (33%) and adolescents (12%) with Bipolar Disorders (Geller et al., 1995). Given the multiple and frequent associations between manic behavior and other difficulties, it is important to consider other possible diagnoses when evaluating the youth who presents with evidence of a Bipolar Disorder.

Quantifying the subjective experience of mood through the use of mood rating scales or other self-report scales can be helpful in monitoring the course of mood disorders. Agreement between child and parent reports are poor for mood disorders (Cantwell, Lewinsohn, Rohde, & Seeley, 1997), and positive reports of symptoms from young people themselves should probably be weighted more heavily than negative reports of symptoms from caretakers. Carlson and Meyer (2006) echo that the assessment of mood is challenging, with poor concordance between parent and child reports, but they remind us that its symptoms should be evident in more than one setting, particularly with symptoms of mania. Explicit questions about the duration, reactivity, and stability of emotional states in children and adolescents can help establish reliable documentation of mood episodes supporting the diagnostic impression of the examiner.

9

Anxiety Problems

OVERVIEW

Anxiety is a ubiquitous human experience, and anxiety symptoms are common in children and adolescents as they react to the familial, social, academic, and personal challenges of development. When nervousness, tension, and other anxiety reactions become more intense, prolonged, and disruptive than typical, the possibility of an Anxiety Disorder or other anxiety-based mental disorder presents itself. Doll's (1996) review of epidemiological studies found Anxiety Disorders to be among the most frequently diagnosed patterns of disturbance in schoolchildren. Our understanding of anxiety problems in young people has advanced appreciably since Miller and colleagues' (1974) seminal discussion, but many remaining issues and controversies continue to make anxiety a perplexing topic. Certain difficulties derive from the nature of the anxiety response itself, whereas others reflect the specific developmental differences between anxiety problems in adults and those in children and adolescents (Birmaher et al., 1997).

The concept of anxiety has been both invaluable and frustrating to many investigators and therapists. Anxiety is a multifaceted construct that can be considered and measured from several perspectives—physiological, behavioral, cognitive, and phenomenological.

Our understanding of the biological basis of anxiety has grown tremendously over the past few decades, with fuller knowledge of the neurological and neurohormonal systems involved in the experience of tension, anxiety, fear, and panic. Multiple physical symptoms are often readily apparent in anxiety reactions: increased striated muscle tension, muscle tremor, changes in perspiration and salivation, increased heart rate, increased blood pressure, temperature changes in the extremities, shifts in stomach acidity and gastric activity, perceptual phenomena associated with increased facial muscle tension, and changes in brain activity have all been investigated. In addition to expanding our understanding of what anxiety is, these physical changes have provided different means of assessing anxiety. Many different physical measures of tension have been developed for laboratory investigations. A potentially significant development was the recognition that various physiological measures of anxiety do not perfectly covary and that a great deal of individual variability exists in different people's responsiveness along different biological channels when presented with anxiety-evoking stimuli. Although our present diagnostic categories remain based on historically recognized patterns of subjectively reported experiences and observed behavioral characteristics, it is quite possible that future diagnostic formulations may be based on different biological systems mediating anxiety responses.

Behavioral or motoric aspects of anxiety involve the typical avoidance or escape behavior seen when an individual is confronted with cues evoking high levels of fear. Intense anxiety is usually an aversive experience, and reduction of fear typically functions as a negative reinforcer. For example, children confronted with a frightening dog next door will run away to escape from it; later they will avoid going into that yard to prevent another encounter with the beast. Successful escape and avoidance are strengthened by the arousal reduction they produce or maintain. A common conceptual formulation of anxiety problems is that they are exaggerated anxiety control responses that are no longer functional. Although escape from actual danger (either physical danger or a threat to self-esteem) is usually adaptive, excessive reactions to overestimated threats tend to cause too much distress or limit effective coping. For example, one of us evaluated an adolescent with a snake phobia who had responded to his roommate throwing a rubber snake at him by scrambling out his second-floor bedroom window. He risked serious physical harm, motivated by a fear he knew to be unrealistic.

The cognitive aspects of anxiety reflect the disruption of higher mental processes seen with elevated tension and arousal. Thinking, abstract reasoning, planning, problem solving, and effective recall are all interfered with by high anxiety. When students report that they really know more than their test scores indicate, there is often a core of truth in their rationalization. Anxiety interferes with cognitive processing. Although many adolescents may maintain that they perform best (or can only perform) under pressure, the weight of the evidence is against this position.

Finally, there is the phenomenological or subjective experience of anxiety that is so familiar to most of us. There is a sense of dread, despair, and impending doom that we cannot control. We may experience sensations of suffocation; fears of impending death; anticipation of unarticulated catastrophe; and loss of control over our breath, swallowing, speech, and coordination. Anxiety is part of human life, and most of us are more familiar than we would care to be with the private experience of this most human emotion. Adolescents, like adults, can easily learn to capture this subjective experience with various reporting devices such as "subjective units of disturbance" (SUDs; Wolpe, 1990), 100-millimeter lines, and other rating scales. Children can usually learn to use age-appropriate analogue reporting methods, such as "fear thermometers."

These aspects of anxiety are not rigidly compartmentalized but fade into each other. For instance, when a student "forgets" about a forthcoming test that he or she has been worried about, is this avoidance a cognitive or a behavioral manifestation? More important than worrying about abstract boundaries is the recognition that anxiety is a complex response with multiple manifestations (i.e., symptoms). Anxiety symptoms occur as part of many psychiatric disorders. Anxiety symptoms are common in depression and other Mood Disorders as well as in Somatoform and Dissociative Disorders, in some Sleep Disorders, and in Substance Use Disorders. In fact, in most of the disorders classified in DSM-5, anxiety symptoms may sometimes occur. But when the anxiety symptoms are the primary manifestations of difficulty, we can conceptualize the problem as a potential Anxiety Disorder (or other anxiety-based mental disorder) and begin looking for characteristic patterns of symptoms—anxiety syndromes such as Panic Attacks or Agoraphobia and other recognized clinical pictures, such as phobias, obsessive–compulsive reactions, or posttraumatic stress reactions. The organizing distinction among "symptoms," "syndromes," and "disorders" is helpful here. Anxiety symptoms are common in all children at different times and circumstances. Anxiety syndromes, clusters of symptoms covarying together, occur less commonly and for varying periods of duration. When an anxiety syndrome persists for some minimal duration and causes either significant personal distress or functional impairment, the essential requirements for an Anxiety Disorder (or other disorder centering around anxiety) are met.

The "Anxiety Disorders" chapter of DSM-5 brings together many of the syndromes and disorders in this classification system in which anxiety symptoms are the primary clinical concern. Additional diagnoses in children and adolescents that, in the past, have been viewed as anxiety-based are included in other related chapters. They are Obsessive–Compulsive Disorder, Reactive Attachment Disorder, Posttraumatic Stress Disorder, Adjustment Disorder with Anxiety, and Avoidant Personality Disorder. A major conceptual shift in DSM-5 has been to separate out situational disorders (Posttraumatic Stress Disorder, Adjustment Disorders) and

Obsessive–Compulsive Disorder into their own chapters. Illness Anxiety Disorder, a new addition to DSM-5, is covered in the "Somatic Symptom and Related Disorders" chapter. A detailed description of the changes in this diagnostic category between editions is provided in the next DSM-IV Note. (We discuss Avoidant Personality Disorder in this chapter in connection with the differential diagnosis of Social Anxiety Disorder; it is discussed further in its own right in Chapter 15.) The IDEA Note on pages 110–111 sets forth how these disorders relate to eligibility for services under IDEA.

SPECIFIC ANXIETY PATTERNS

As would be expected, DSM-5 approaches Anxiety Disorders (and other related disorders) by identifying a variety of specific symptom groupings that have been recognized in clinical practice. The broad heuristic for the evaluator is, first, the recognition that many or most of a child's or adolescent's problems can be conceptualized as anxiety difficulties; second, the exclusion of more pervasive problems for which anxiety can be an associated symptom (general medical conditions, Psychotic Disorders, Mood Disorders); and, third, the identification of the specific pattern or patterns of symptoms most characteristic of the young person's problems. The issue of a more pervasive disorder's preempting the diagnosis of less global disorders is important in the assessment and diagnosis of Anxiety Disorders. Anxiety as a symptom is common in many emotional and behavioral disorders; only when it is the core of the difficulty is an Anxiety Disorder diagnosed. An Anxiety Disorder can be diagnosed concurrently with a Mood Disorder such as Major Depressive Disorder, but only when there is evidence that the Anxiety Disorder is a separate problem. For instance, if the child has a history of a clinical Phobia for several years and (while this problem continues) then develops Major Depressive Disorder, both diagnoses should be made. This example illustrates the basic situation of diagnosing two disorders when one is an associated symptom of the other: In this case, there is evidence of independent occurrence of the two dysfunctions.

The "Anxiety Disorders" chapter of DSM-5 begins with Separation Anxiety Disorder. This disorder is a new addition to the chapter on anxiety disorders, moved to appear as the first category in the "Anxiety Disorders" chapter because it is the earliest appearing disorder reflecting disturbances involving fear, anxiety, and/or avoidance.

Separation Anxiety Disorder

Separation Anxiety Disorder is one of the more frequent clinical anxiety presentations in children (Suveg, Aschenbrand, & Kendall, 2005) and is

DSM-IV Note. Changes in DSM-5 for Anxiety and Related Disorders

The structure and order of presentation of anxiety disorders in DSM-5 differs from that provided by DSM-IV. One notable change is that Separation Anxiety Disorder and Selective Mutism, formerly housed in "Disorders Usually First Diagnosed in Infancy, Childhood, and Adolescence," have joined the "Anxiety Disorders" chapter in DSM-5. Several other disorders formerly included in the chapter on anxiety disorders in DSM-IV have been partitioned into other free-standing chapters, including Posttraumatic Stress Disorder, Reactive Attachment Disorder, and Disinhibited Social Engagement Disorder, in the new "Trauma and Stressor-Related Disorders" chapter, and Obsessive–Compulsive Disorder, Body Dysmorphic Disorder, Hoarding Disorder, Trichotillomania (Hair-Pulling Disorder), and Excoriation (Skin-Picking) Disorder in the new "Obsessive–Compulsive and Related Disorders" chapter. One final disorder, Illness Anxiety Disorder, new to DSM, is located in the "Somatic Symptom and Related Disorders" chapter and captures distressed reactions to medical conditions that interfere with functioning (see further discussion of this disorder in the "Somatic Symptom and Related Disorders" section in Chapter 10 in this volume). Within the "Anxiety Disorders" chapter, the disorders are presented in order of developmental appearance. That is, they are ordered to reflect their respective typical age of onset, with Separation Anxiety Disorder presented first as the typical earliest-appearing anxiety disorder, followed by Selective Mutism, Specific Phobia, Social Anxiety Disorder, Panic Disorder, Agoraphobia, Generalized Anxiety Disorder, Substance/Medication-Induced Anxiety Disorder, Anxiety Disorder Due to Another Medical Condition, Other Specified Anxiety Disorder, and Unspecified Anxiety Disorder.

In terms of diagnostic criteria for the anxiety disorders, much remains the same, yet several important differences were noted. For some disorders, the criteria were merely reorganized, whereas for others items were added and/or removed. Here are some of the highlights of the changes by disorder.

Separation Anxiety Disorder

The biggest change is the removal of the requisite that onset occur before 18 years of age. Thus this diagnosis is now permissible for adults, but examiners are encouraged to look for a pattern of avoidance, anxiety, or fear symptoms for 6 months, though flexibility is permitted in this criterion. In contrast, these symptoms must only be evident for 4 weeks in children and adolescents.

Selective Mutism

The category of Selective Mutism was added to the "Anxiety Disorders" chapter. No changes were made to its criteria.

Specific Phobia

The language in the DSM-5 is similar to that seen in DSM-IV-TR, but it is not identical. It has also been reorganized, and a few other changes have been made. Specifically, the criteria refer to "fear or anxiety," not just one or the other. The phrase "out of proportion to actual danger" replaces "excessive and unreasonable" (p. 449). In the previous edition, age-based adjustments were made in that children might not recognize that the fear is unreasonable or excessive, but they were required to show evidence of symptoms for at least 6 months. In the current edition, these age-based adjustments are extended to individuals of all ages. In other words, the criteria that the "fear, anxiety, or avoidance is persistent, typically lasting 6 months or more" (p. 197) applies to everyone, not just children, and the requirement that adults recognize that the anxiety is excessive and unreasonable was also removed. The criteria are also less specific about the magnitude of interference in functioning that is required for diagnosis. DSM-5 includes the same five Phobic Stimulus specifiers, and it provides guidance for applying ICD-10 codes for each of them, unlike its predecessor.

Social Anxiety Disorder

Social Anxiety Disorder was referred to as Social Phobia in DSM-IV-TR. This label is provided parenthetically in DSM-5. Many of the changes to Social Anxiety Disorder are similar to the updates for Specific Phobia. That is, the content is similar to its predecessor, but the language was altered and the criteria were reorganized. Like the criteria for Specific Phobia, the symptoms of Social Anxiety Disorder need to be persistent (i.e., 6 months or more), out of proportion, and cause significant distress. The first criterion includes "fear or anxiety," not just fear, as was presented in DSM-IV-TR. They removed the requirements that the individual recognizes that the fear is excessive and that children show evidence of capacity for age-appropriate social relationships. Performance anxiety is also addressed in a slightly different way. Specifically, they moved references to performance to the examples and included Performance Only as a specifier for the disorder. In contrast, DSM-IV-TR only specified Generalized, which is not included as a specifier in DSM-5.

Panic Disorder and Agoraphobia

In DSM-5, Panic Disorder and Agoraphobia are presented separately, unlike in its predecessor, which offered two options: Panic Disorder With Agoraphobia and Panic Disorder Without Agoraphobia. Criterion B for Panic Disorder also combines two separate listings from DSM-IV-TR.

Agoraphobia was formerly described in relation to Panic Disorder or other disorders, but it appears as a separate disorder in DSM-5. Diagnosis requires "marked fear or anxiety" in at least two of five specific situations, namely "using public transportation, being in open spaces, being in enclosed spaces, standing in line or being in a crowd, and being outside of the home alone" (p. 217). The remaining criteria require that the individual almost always experiences out-of-proportion fear or anxiety for 6 months or longer that causes clinically significant distress or impairment. It may be diagnosed with another medical condition if it is excessive for the typical presentation of the other condition.

Generalized Anxiety Disorder

The diagnostic criteria for Generalized Anxiety Disorder have been slightly reorganized, but are essentially the same as in DSM-IV-TR.

Substance/Medication-Induced Anxiety Disorder

DSM-IV-TR included obsessions and compulsions in the diagnostic criteria; DSM-5 does not. DSM-5 also removed the specifiers about anxiety symptoms (e.g., With Generalized Anxiety, With Panic Attacks, With Obsessive-Compulsive Symptoms, With Phobic Symptoms). The specifiers about onset (i.e., With Onset During Intoxication, With Onset During Withdrawal) remain along with one addition: With Onset After Medication Use.

Anxiety Disorder Due to Another Medical Condition

Similar to Substance/Medication-Induced Anxiety Disorder, this category included obsessions and compulsions in DSM-IV-TR, but it does not in DSM-5. It also included specifiers about anxiety symptoms that DSM-5 does not have.

IDEA Note. Anxiety-Related Mental Disorders and IDEA

A diagnosis of an Anxiety Disorder (or other mental disorder centering around anxiety) can form the basis of qualifying a child for special services under the "serious emotional disturbance" or simply "emotional disturbance" category of IDEA. One of the identified conditions indicating "serious emotional disturbance" is a "tendency to develop physical symptoms or fears associated with personal or school problems" that persists "over a long period of time and to a marked degree that adversely affects educational performance" (Individuals with Disabilities Education Improvement Act [IDEA], 2004, Public Law 108-446, paragraph (c)(4)(i)). Severe anxiety symptoms can easily be construed as falling within this condition. Another identified condition is "an inability to build or maintain satisfactory relationships with peers and teachers," which can be a symptom associated with anxiety problems in children and adolescents. Documentation of the functional impairment in academic or social adjustment caused by the anxiety problem will be important. Beyond a formal diagnosis, providing additional information detailing related psychosocial and environmental considerations and the child's functioning may also be important in establishing eligibility for services under IDEA.

The IDEA requirement that the qualifying condition must have a negative influence on educational performance opens the possibility of conundrums in the application of the IDEA system versus the DSM system. It is possible that a child or adolescent might be miserable and show significant social maladjustment but maintain acceptable school performance. This young person, even though manifesting a severe Anxiety Disorder or other related disorder, might not be eligible for services under IDEA. Much more typical, however, is obvious impairment in academic achievement associated with severe anxiety symptoms.

One complication of evaluating Anxiety Disorders and other anxiety problems, especially in children, is that many of the manifestations may be largely in the nature of private experience. Children may be acutely distressed by their fear, worry, and tension; however, unless they report these experiences, act it out in behavioral avoidance/escape, or exhibit a clearly disrupted level of performance in academic or everyday tasks, teachers, parents, or other caretakers may remain unaware of the children's suffering. The difficulties inherent in evaluating private experiences, especially in younger children, necessitate that examiners aggressively explore reports or behaviors suggesting anxiety problems in children and make use of multiple sources of data. Indications from the young persons themselves of problems with anxiety should be weighted more heavily than negative reports from caretakers (Cantwell et al., 1997). While remaining cognizant of the reality that fears and even extreme fears are common and usually transient in children, a school psychologist also needs to be sensitive to indications that anxiety phenomena are enduring in a child's life; are causing a great deal of unhappiness; or are contributing to failures in expected personal, social, or academic development. Our impression is that anxiety problems are underdiagnosed in school-age children. Adults often fail to recognize their problems or misattribute them to the "normal" vicissitudes of growing up.

---

one of the few anxiety-related mental disorders for which there is reasonable congruence between child and caretaker reports (Cantwell et al., 1997). The key feature in the accurate diagnosis of Separation Anxiety Disorder is that a child's separation from his or her primary caretaker serves as the effective stimulus for the intense anxiety reaction. It is seen in situations in which the child is being left off at day care or school by the caretaker or when the child is left home with a babysitter and the caretaker leaves; it is usually quickly relieved by reunion with the caretaker. The child may have problems being apart from the caretaker even within the home (e.g., unwillingness to sleep in his or her own bed). The relationship of this disorder to earlier, developmentally normal fears (fear of strangers, developmentally typical separation anxiety) is of continuing interest.

School avoidance or refusal is reported as a symptom of Separation Anxiety Disorder in the majority of cases (approximately 75%, according to Francis, Last, & Strauss, 1987); however, some care should be taken to evaluate and eliminate the possibility that the fear response is to some stimulus element in the situation (i.e., fear of school or some aspect of school vs. fear of separation from the caretaker). The evaluator should also keep in mind that separation anxiety is common and normal in younger children. Nevertheless, it is important to evaluate the intensity and quality of a child's separation anxiety experience and its effects upon his or her adjustment. Separation Anxiety Disorder *is* a Mental Disorder—the anxiety about separation from caretakers is excessive and maladaptive.

Selective Mutism

Selective Mutism (Elective Mutism in DSM-III and DSM-III-R) has also been referred to as "voluntary silence." Selective Mutism is a rare disorder. The key feature of selective mutism is the lack of speech in the presence of others when the ability to communicate verbally has been established in other contexts. Thus the child in question is able to talk (documented by observation in other settings) but chooses not to in at least one specific social setting, causing social or educational problems. This diagnosis presents as an interesting pattern that often manifests itself primarily in the school setting. A frequent presentation of selective mutism involves a school-age child who willingly converses with family and friends at home but does not speak at school when a teacher and/or others are present.

Although in the past Selective Mutism was often discussed in the context of communication difficulties, approximately two-thirds of children with Selective Mutism have no other unusual speech characteristics. The problem appears to be more of an emotional or behavioral disturbance than a communication difficulty. This disorder is conceptualized as anxiety-driven, explaining its placement in the "Anxiety Disorders" chapter. This view is supported by research (e.g., Dummit et al., 1997) indicating that this disorder usually presents in the context of Anxiety Disorders. Steinhausen and Juzi (1996) reported that shyness and internalizing behavior problems were the most frequent personality features noted in a series of 100 cases of DSM-III-R Elective Mutism. Selective Mutism may be comorbid with Social Phobia, and both disorders should be diagnosed in such a case. A population study covering two school districts in Sweden found a higher prevalence rate than had been previously estimated—approximately 18 cases per 10,000 children ages 7–15 years (Kopp & Gillberg, 1997). A more recent study estimated Selective Mutism to affect between 0.03 and 0.2% of children and adolescents (Carbone et al., 2010). The association of Selective Mutism with social reticence, possibly in the parents as well as the child, may act to suppress detection and awareness of this problem (Kopp & Gillberg, 1997).

Assessment requires the examiner to gather data from multiple informants, including teachers, parents or guardians, peers, and siblings. Differentiating Selective Mutism from shyness, an autism spectrum disorder, and other anxiety disorders requires careful attention to interviews with knowledgeable informants. The main symptom of Selective Mutism (i.e., not speaking) has the potential to interfere with school performance, particularly in classes that require presentations or other verbal participation. Beyond academic performance, Selective Mutism can also affect social functioning and peer relationships. If either or both of these areas of functioning are impaired, it could be reason to consider eligibility for special education services under the category of "Serious Emotional Disturbance."

Panic Disorder

A panic attack is an episode of intense fear, physiological arousal, and (often) frantic escape behavior, occurring during a discrete period of time (i.e., peaking within 10 minutes). Panic attacks are not a codable disorder in their own right; they occur in the context of another condition. When these attacks are followed by at least a month of worry or problematic change in behavior, an individual may meet the criteria for Panic Disorder. It is also possible that an individual presents with another anxiety, mental, or medical condition along with panic attacks, in which case the specifier, "With Panic Attacks" would be applied.

Panic attacks are sufficiently distinct from normal experience and noxious in character that adult clients usually give relatively clear and reliable accounts of their occurrence. Panic attacks in children have received some discussion in the literature, but little is clear. It is not certain how frequent this experience is prior to adolescence, or even whether it occurs at all prior to puberty (Bernstein & Borchardt, 1991). A study by Biederman and colleagues (1997) suggests that Panic Disorder and Agoraphobia may occur with some frequency in clinical populations but may not be easily recognized. Research on panic attacks in both clinical (Kearney, Albano, Eisen, Allan, & Barlow, 1997) and nonclinical (Hayward et al., 1997) populations of youth are beginning to provide a more empirical foundation of knowledge on this subject.

Agoraphobia

Agoraphobia is a frequently seen fear syndrome in adult clinical settings, but it appears to be infrequent in children and adolescents. A commonly offered model of Agoraphobia sees it as usually, but not inevitably, associated with a history of cued or uncued panic attacks; Agoraphobia is an acute fear of being in circumstances in which the person may be unable to escape or get help if the need arises. Agoraphobia is thought of as a "fear of fear," or catastrophic misinterpretation of physiological cues of increasing tension. Although this view is appealing, it may not be consistent with the empirical data on the relative prevalence of panic attacks and Agoraphobia and their respective ages of onset (Biederman et al., 1997). Many empirical and theoretical questions remain to be resolved regarding these two syndromes.

Although panic attacks and Agoraphobia may be useful in conceptualizing adult anxiety problems, in our experiences they have limited application to juvenile situations. The remaining Anxiety Disorders are relatively frequent in children and adolescents, as is one of the Adjustment Disorder diagnoses focused on anxiety symptoms.

Specific Phobias

Fears are common in children, and even intense fears occur with some frequency (Gullone, 2000; Milne et al., 1995). By contrast, a "phobia" has been defined as a "special form of fear" that is excessive, maladaptive, persistent, and (in the case of children) "not age or state specific" (Marks, 1969, quoted in Miller et al., 1974, p. 90). Mild fears are common and usually transient; severe fears are more likely to continue over time; and phobias tend to be stable without systematic intervention. The intensity and predictability of the anxiety reaction to the identified phobic stimulus usually make diagnosis fairly straightforward. Phobia-like elements make up part of the clinical picture of Obsessive–Compulsive Disorder and Posttraumatic Stress Disorder, as well as of Specific Phobias and Social Phobia.

More so than the other anxiety disorders, Specific Phobias—intense, stable fears of discrete situations or objects—can and do occur in isolation from other anxiety or depressive difficulties. Phobias involving blood or injury, for instance, have usually been reported without significant rates of comorbidities (Marks, 1988). If there is a fear of phobic intensity, however, the majority of cases will show other extreme fears (Milne et al., 1995). The important element of a Specific Phobia is the exaggerated anxiety response relative to any degree of actual physical or psychological risk present in the situation, which leads to maladaptive responding. Five phobic stimuli may be specified in DSM-5: Animal, Natural Environment, Blood-Injection-Injury, Situational, or Other. When more than one specific phobia is present, codes are provided for each.

Social Anxiety Disorder (Social Phobia)

When a phobic reaction is elicited by interpersonal stimuli, the diagnosis of Social Anxiety Disorder is made. Youth with Social Phobia show extreme anxiety in situations in which they feel evaluated by others; they fear being embarrassed, humiliated, or thought poorly of by other people. In some cases, this may center around a particular concern (e.g., blushing). One young adolescent one of us consulted with could barely stand being looked at by others because of her fear that she would blush and they would laugh at her. Alternatively, the fear may be a general sense of looking "stupid," saying something "dumb," or being found generally lacking in some undefined way. Whereas social anxieties are relatively common in adolescents and adults, Social Anxiety Disorder can be conceptualized as an extreme point on a dimension of concern about social evaluation. Its onset is usually in adolescence (Herbert, 1995), and without treatment the course is often chronic, with significant personal, social, and vocational impairment. There is frequent comorbidity with other anxiety disorders and depression, as well as an increased risk of substance abuse (Herbert, 1995).

The diagnosis of Social Anxiety Disorder in children and adolescents brings up boundary issues with Avoidant Personality Disorder, which are difficult to resolve within the directives given by DSM-5. Both diagnoses focus on anxiety symptoms elicited by interpersonal exposure and interaction. The overlap in defining symptoms yields very high comorbidities. Avoidant Personality Disorder occurs in 25–70% of clients diagnosed with Social Anxiety Disorder, and Social Anxiety Disorder can almost always be diagnosed in clients with Avoidant Personality Disorder (Herbert, 1995). These two categories are probably not distinct phenomenological or symptomatic clusters (Francis, Last, & Strauss, 1992). Avoidant Personality Disorder may well represent a more severe manifestation of the same basic pattern reflected in Social Anxiety Disorder. Given the thorny conceptual issues in considering a Personality Disorder with adolescents and especially children (see Chapter 15), we recommend that the category of Social Anxiety Disorder be used when the differential diagnosis is between this category and Avoidant Personality Disorder in children.

"School phobia" is not a diagnosis available within DSM-5. Bernstein and Borchardt (1991) suggest that in a high percentage of cases of school refusal, separation anxiety is found to be manifested, and that many of these children may meet criteria for Separation Anxiety Disorder (see earlier in this chapter). Some children, however, present with a distinct fear of school rather than Separation Anxiety Disorder and are probably best conceptualized as having a variant of Social Anxiety Disorder (Last, Francis, Hersen, Kazdin, & Strauss, 1987). Like young people with other anxiety problems, youth with school avoidance or refusal may not acknowledge that their fears are excessive or unreasonable. Symptoms of school avoidance or refusal may also occur in the cluster of conduct problems in which they reflect not anxiety but self-indulgence. For treatment planning, the important differential diagnosis is between school avoidance as a manifestation of an Anxiety Disorder and school avoidance as a manifestation of a Disruptive Behavior Disorder.

Generalized Anxiety Disorder

Generalized Anxiety Disorder involves a grouping of anxiety symptoms and worry that occur without specific eliciting stimuli. The individual shows a pervasive and enduring pattern of excessive arousal. This pattern in children was previously labeled Overanxious Disorder of Childhood until it was formally acknowledged in DSM-IV that the child, adolescent, and adult manifestations are essentially identical. Excessive worry ("apprehensive expectation") is a defining feature of Generalized Anxiety Disorder that is certainly consistent with the clinical literature on children (Strauss, Lease, Last, & Francis, 1988). High comorbidities are reported with other anxiety disorders, depression, and Attention-Deficit/Hyperactivity Disorder—a pattern of comorbidity seen for many anxiety disorders in children, as noted earlier.

Other Specific Categories within Anxiety Disorders

Anxiety Disorders in children and adolescents can develop as a consequence of substance use (Substance/Medication-Induced Anxiety Disorder) or a general medical condition (Anxiety Disorder Due to Another Medical Condition). That is, generalized nervousness and tension, fears, panic attacks, or obsessive–compulsive symptoms may develop during drug or medication intoxication or withdrawal, as well as in response to illness, injury, or some other physiological influence. Anxiety problems may also develop that do not conform to any of the specific symptom patterns identified (Other Specified or Unspecified Anxiety Disorder).

OBSESSIVE–COMPULSIVE AND RELATED DISORDERS

DSM-5 moved Obsessive–Compulsive Disorder out of the chapter on anxiety disorders to lead a separate chapter of related disorders. These categories include Obsessive–Compulsive Disorder, Body Dysmorphic Disorder, Hoarding Disorder, Trichotillomania, Excoriation, Substance/Medication-Induced Obsessive–Compulsive and Related Disorder, Obsessive–Compulsive and Related Disorder Due to Another Medical Condition, Other Specified Obsessive–Compulsive and Related Disorder, and Unspecified Obsessive–Compulsive and Related Disorder. Although Obsessive–Compulsive Disorder and its related disorders are now presented in a separate chapter, the authors of DSM-5 acknowledge the "close relationships between the anxiety disorders and some of the obsessive–compulsive and related disorders (e.g., Obsessive–Compulsive Disorder), which is reflected in the sequence of DSM-5 chapters" (p. 235). A detailed list of changes to the diagnostic criteria for disorders in this category from the previous edition is provided in the next DSM-IV-TR Note.

DSM-IV-TR Note. Changes in DSM-5 for Obsessive–Compulsive and Related Disorders

The biggest change is the location of these disorders in their own freestanding chapter positioned near but not within the Anxiety Disorders chapter. Changes to specific disorders within this chapter are described in this note.

Obsessive–Compulsive Disorder

The requirement that the obsessions are not simply excessive worries about real-world problems was removed. The individual also does not have to recognize that the obsessions are a product of his or her own mind. Specifiers were also added to this diagnosis for insight (i.e., With Good or Fair Insight; With Poor Insight; With Absent Insight/Delusional Beliefs) and past or present comorbid Tic Disorder.

Body Dysmorphic Disorder

The new criteria require that the individual has at some point performed repetitive behaviors related to concerns about appearance. It also includes several specifiers for insight (identical to those listed for Obsessive–Compulsive Disorder) and focused on the quality of the individual's body build (i.e., With Muscle Dysmorphia).

Trichotillomania

Unlike DSM-IV-TR, the DSM-5 criteria require that the hair loss be noticeable. It also requires that the individual make repeated attempts to eliminate or reduce hair pulling. DSM-IV-TR required a sense of tension tied to pulling or resisting pulling hair and pleasure, gratification, or relief upon doing so; DSM-5 does not require any of these symptoms.

All of the remaining disorders in this chapter are new in DSM-5. These disorders include Hoarding Disorder, Excoriation (Skin-Picking) Disorder, Substance/Medication-Induced Obsessive–Compulsive and Related Disorder, Obsessive–Compulsive and Related Disorder Due to Another Medical Condition, Other Specified Obsessive–Compulsive and Related Disorder, and Unspecified Obsessive–Compulsive and Related Disorder.

Obsessive–Compulsive Disorder

Obsessive–Compulsive Disorder has been increasingly acknowledged as more common in children and adolescents than previously believed, although failure to recognize these problems continues (March & Leonard, 1996). Young people with Obsessive–Compulsive Disorder are often sensitive to the negative reactions of others and may carry out their compulsive behaviors in secret. A child or adolescent may come to the attention of the school psychologist because of secondary problems—academic difficulties caused by obsessive concerns and ritualistic behavior, a teacher's concern over frequent requests to be excused to the washroom, or physical signs of excessive washing (Adams, Waas, March, & Smith, 1994). Common obsessions and compulsions reported in child clinical cases by March and Leonard (1996) are shown in Table 9.1. Washing and checking rituals are reported to occur in most child cases at some point in the clinical course (Swedo, Rapoport, Leonard, Lenane, & Cheslow, 1989).

Although either intrusive thoughts or ritualistic behaviors will satisfy the diagnostic requirements, both types of features are usually seen in clinical cases. The behavior must cause the young person distress, take up excessive amounts of time, or interfere with functional adjustment (school performance, social activities, or important relationships). Children do not need to recognize the illogical nature of their behavior (though they usually do); With Poor Insight or With Absent Insight/Delusional Beliefs may be noted if there is not some acknowledgment of the excessive and senseless nature of the symptoms or if the child is convinced that the Obsessive–Compulsive Disorder beliefs are true, respectively.

TABLE 9.1. Common Obsessions and Compulsions Reported in Child Cases

Obsessions	Compulsions
Contamination themes	Washing
Harm to self or others	Repeating
Aggressive themes	Checking
Sexual themes	Touching
Scrupulosity/religiosity	Counting
Forbidden thoughts	Ordering/arranging
Symmetry urges	Hoarding
Need to tell, ask, confess	Praying

Note. From March and Leonard (1996). Copyright 1996 by the American Academy of Child and Adolescent Psychiatry. Reprinted by permission.

Other Anxiety Disorders are often seen in children with Obsessive–Compulsive Disorder (especially Specific Phobias, Social Anxiety Disorder, and Generalized Anxiety Disorder). Tic Disorders (including Tourette's Disorder) have been found to be associated with Obsessive–Compulsive Disorder in some families (March & Leonard, 1996; Pauls, Alsobrook, Goodman, Rasmussen, & Leckman, 1995). Disruptive Behavior Disorders and Learning Disorders are reported to be common associated problems of children with Obsessive–Compulsive Disorder; obsessive–compulsive-related disorders (i.e., Trichotillomania, Body Dysmorphic Disorder, and habit problems such as nail biting) are said to occur as less frequent comorbidities (March & Leonard, 1996). In particular, Obsessive–Compulsive Disorder and Tourette's Disorder appear in at least some instances to be alternative phenotypical expressions of a common genotype (March & Leonard, 1996). The report of an association among Obsessive–Compulsive Disorder, Tourette's Disorder, and a trait marker of streptococcal infections will no doubt intensify the search for a possible neurological foundation for these disorders (Swedo et al., 1997).

Obsessive–Compulsive Disorder and Obsessive–Compulsive Personality Disorder, despite the similarity of their titles, do not appear to covary at any meaningful frequency in children or adolescents.

DISORDERS DISCUSSED ALONG WITH OBSESSIVE–COMPULSIVE DISORDER

As noted before, several other disorders are included with Obsessive–Compulsive Disorder in the new chapter. These are Body Dysmorphic Disorder (grouped in DSM-IV with Somatoform Disorders), Hoarding Disorder, Trichotillomania, Excoriation Disorder, the Substance/Medication Induced and Due to Another Medical Condition, and residual categories, Other Specified and Unspecified.

Body Dysmorphic Disorder

Body Dysmorphic Disorder, or "dysmorphophobia" as it has traditionally been called in the literature, reflects a preoccupation with some perceived deficit in physical appearance (e.g., nose too large, breasts too small, inadequate musculature). The concern is intense enough to cause significant personal distress or functional impairment (i.e., it meets criteria for a Mental Disorder). The onset of Body Dysmorphic Disorder is probably during adolescence, but most known cases involve adults. Careful review of how much time is spent per day ruminating about or inspecting the offending body part(s), evaluation of the presence and intensity of anxiety symptoms, and especially assessment of avoidance behavior or social withdrawal because of the perceived "deformity" are useful in establishing a clinical diagnosis. DSM-5 notes the higher associated suicide risk, greater comorbidity, and typically gradual onset in clients with onset of this disorder prior to age 18. Risk factors include a history of childhood neglect and abuse, as well as first-degree relatives with diagnoses of an Obsessive–Compulsive Disorder.

Hoarding Disorder

Hoarding Disorder is a new diagnostic category in DSM-5. The text reports that this problem tends to begin in adolescence (11–15 years of age) and exacerbates to clinical severity through interference with functional behavior during the client's 20s, with increasing severity often accruing over the lifespan. Little empirical information is available on this disorder in youth.

Trichotillomania (Hair-Pulling Disorder)

Trichotillomania (Hair-Pulling Disorder) has long been recognized as a low-prevalence behavior disorder. The text notes that this behavior may be seen in infants but typically comes under fairly rapid control. Clinical cases show continued problems with high frequency and/or recurrent episodes of hair pulling. Clinical cases of Trichotillomania are seen in children as well as adolescents and adults. The most well-established risk factor appears to be concurrent Obsessive–Compulsive Disorder and/or having first-degree relatives with Obsessive–Compulsive Disorder. In youth, we have that seen Trichotillomania is sometimes associated with trichophagia (a form of Pica in which hair is eaten). We have also noted an interesting dichotomy between cases in which the hair pulling is conscious, deliberate, and usually associated with a perception of an increasing and aversive internal sensation that is relieved by the act and cases in which the behavior seems to occur more "unconsciously," automatically, and unintentionally while the individual is focused on other activities, such as reading or watching television. Our clinical samples are too limited to be confident of treatment differentials with these two different patterns. Flessner (2011) gives a review of cognitive-behavioral treatments for repetitive disorders in children, including Trichotillomania; Bloch, Panza, Grant, Pittenger, and Leckman (2013) found no benefit for *N*-acetylcystein in the treatment of Trichotillomania in children despite a report of positive results in adults. Much further research is needed on all of the associated disorders in this group.

Excoriation (Skin-Picking) Disorder

Excoriation (Skin-Picking) Disorder is another new DSM-5 diagnosis, and the empirical literature on this problem, especially in youth, is limited. The text notes the association with Obsessive–Compulsive Disorder and Trichotillomania, as well as Major Depressive Disorder. The text also notes that other repetitive body-focused symptoms may occur in individuals with Excoriation Disorder and that, if they cause significant distress or functional impairment, they may warrant an additional diagnosis of Other Specified Obsessive–Compulsive and Related Disorder: Body Focused and Repetitive Behavior Disorder. This example illustrates one use of the Other Specified categories, which is to identify problematic behaviors related to but different from designated diagnoses. We have also seen skin picking as a self-injurious behavior in individuals with Borderline Personality Disorder. In most of those instances the skin picking is viewed as an associated symptom of the Borderline Personality Disorder and is not diagnosed separately.

TRAUMA- AND STRESSOR-RELATED DISORDERS

In addition to a new, separate chapter covering Obsessive–Compulsive and Related Disorders, the authors of DSM-5 removed Posttraumatic Stress Disorder from the "Anxiety Disorders" chapter and placed it in a new chapter containing Trauma- and Stressor-Related Disorders. This chapter includes Reactive Attachment Disorder (formerly in the chapter on Disorders Usually First Diagnosed in Infancy, Childhood, or Adolescence), Disinhibited Social Engagement Disorder (new disorder), Posttraumatic Stress Disorder, Acute Stress Disorder, and Adjustment Disorders (formerly in their own chapter). These disorders are clustered together because they all require exposure to a specific traumatic or stressful event as a criterion. Changes to these disorders in DSM-5 are provided in the next DSM-IV-TR Note.

Disorders Related to the Caregiving Relationship

Both Reactive Attachment Disorder and Disinhibited Social Engagement Disorder are conceptualized as disorders stemming from a lack of adequate caregiving. Internalizing symptoms of an underlying attachment dysfunction are captured by a diagnosis of Reactive Attachment Disorder, whereas externalizing symptoms of an attachment deficit are captured in the new DSM-5 diagnosis of Disinhibited Social Engagement Disorder. These disorders were both formerly considered Reactive Attachment Disorder in

DSM-IV Note. Changes in DSM-5 for Trauma- and Stressor-Related Disorders

Reactive Attachment Disorder

Now appearing in the "Trauma- and Stressor-Related Disorders" chapter, Reactive Attachment Disorder in DSM-IV-TR has been divided into two separate disorders in DSM-5: Reactive Attachment Disorder and Disinhibited Social Engagement Disorder. Although the diagnostic label of the former is the same, the criteria are quite different and center on nonengagement with caregivers and lack of positive emotions. The new criteria require both minimal or absent comfort-seeking from and responsiveness to the caregiver. It is characterized as a "persistent social and emotional disturbance" (p. 265) that includes at least two of three symptoms: minimal responsiveness to others, limited positive affect, and episodes of irritability, sadness, or fearfulness. Importantly, lack of adequate caregiving must be accountable for the symptoms. That is, the child must present with a history of severe neglect, multiple changes in primary caregiver without adequate opportunity to form attachment, or inadequate opportunities to form attachments.

DSM-IV-TR required onset before age 5. This requisite is maintained in DSM-5 with the addition of an onset floor: It must be evident after 9 months of age. The specifiers for Reactive Attachment Disorder have also changed. Examiners now indicate whether the disorder is persistent (i.e., lasting for more than 12 months) and/or severe (i.e., child exhibits all symptoms). It is also noteworthy that indiscriminant sociability was eliminated as a criterion for Reactive Attachment Disorder. It now forms the basis of the Disinhibited Social Engagement Disorder diagnosis.

Disinhibited Social Engagement Disorder

New to DSM-5, Disinhibited Social Engagement Disorder captures the overly familiar and indiscriminant interactions with others that were formerly included in Reactive Attachment Disorder. The underlying cause (i.e., lack of adequate caregiving) is thought to be the same for these two disorders; however, the presentation differs, with internalizing symptoms present in children with Reactive Attachment Disorder and externalizing behavior present in children with Disinhibited Social Engagement Disorder.

Posttraumatic Stress Disorder

One major change from DSM-IV-TR is that DSM-5 provides separate criteria for individuals under the age of 6. Also new to DSM-5 are two additional possibilities of exposure to the traumatic event, namely learning that a traumatic event occurred to a family member or close friend and repeated or extreme exposure to the specifics of the traumatic event. DSM-IV-TR required that the individual respond with intense fear, helplessness, or horror. In contrast, DSM-5 does not include this criterion. The diagnostic criteria are also divided differently, requiring the presence of at least one symptom within the following categories: intrusion, avoidance, changes in cognitions and mood, and changes in arousal and reactivity. The specifiers in DSM-5 are also different. Examiners are to indicate whether dissociative symptoms are present. If so, they are to indicate the presence of depersonalization and derealization. The specifier "With Delayed Expression," replaces "With Delayed Onset" to indicate onset of meeting the full diagnostic criteria 6 months or more after exposure to the stressor. Criteria for children under age 6 are adjusted somewhat to account for developmental expectations. For example, children under age 6 need only demonstrate either avoidance or changes in mood and/or cognition; these criteria are combined for children under 6 years old.

Acute Stress Disorder

Acute Stress Disorder was new to DSM-IV. In DSM-5, the diagnostic criteria evidence a few important changes for this disorder. Similar to the changes in Posttraumatic Stress Disorder, the criteria for Acute Stress Disorder detail two additional methods of exposure to traumatic event(s), and they no longer require that the individual respond to the traumatic event(s) with fear, helplessness, or terror. Diagnosis now requires the presence of nine or more symptoms clustered into five categories: intrusion symptoms, negative mood, dissociative symptoms, avoidance symptoms, and arousal symptoms. Another major change from DSM-IV-TR is the shift away from requiring symptoms of dissociation. That is, DSM-IV-TR required three or more symptoms of dissociation, whereas DSM-5 requires nine or more symptoms, some of which may, but do not have to, be dissociative.

DSM-IV-TR. We recommend great care in assigning these diagnoses. The literature on attachment problems is mixed with evidence of conceptual confusion and of cases that lack compelling documentation of the presumptive pathological care required for the diagnosis. Even with clear evidence of severe neglect, the examiner cannot automatically assume an attachment disorder. See Woolgar and Scott (2014) for a discussion of these topics.

Posttraumatic Stress Disorder

Posttraumatic Stress Disorder involves a triad of defining symptoms following exposure to an extremely traumatic stressor. The core symptoms are (1) a recurrent reexperiencing of the stressor, (2) persistent avoidance of reminders of the event and a decrease in general responsiveness ("numbing"), and (3) persistent hyperarousal. Some amount of controversy has surrounded this diagnosis since its introduction in DSM-III, but overall both the clinical experience of practitioners and the empirical literature appear to support its basic validity and utility. Critical concerns about the accurate diagnosis of Posttraumatic Stress Disorder center on three issues, which are discussed in this section: (1) the nature of the stressful event, (2) the defining pattern of symptoms, and (3) the course of the disorder. Important additional topics beyond the scope of this discussion include the possibility of individual differences or premorbid risk factors that may predispose children to develop Posttraumatic Stress Disorder and possible neurological changes underlying Posttraumatic Stress Disorder. It is worth noting that Posttraumatic Stress Disorder is one of the very few disorders for which DSM-5 specifies etiological circumstances.

The Nature of the Traumatic Stress

DSM-III and DSM-III-R built the category of Posttraumatic Stress Disorder around the concept of a psychologically disturbing event that is beyond the range of typical human experience. This notion proved troublesome in application and was ultimately rejected as unworkable. In its Criterion A for Posttraumatic Stress Disorder, DSM-IV replaced this formulation with a specification of a traumatic event that has two defining features: (1) There is exposure to the risk or actuality of death, serious harm, or loss of physical integrity and (2) the client's reaction includes either intense negative emotion (fear, horror, helplessness) or (in children) disorganized behavior or agitation. In DSM-5, the diagnostic criteria for this disorder no longer require the second feature (i.e., the response of intense negative emotion); however, it does require the combination of exposure to a traumatic event and symptoms of intrusion, avoidance, changes in cognition and mood, and arousal/reactivity. These changes provide a serviceable conceptualization of the circumstances that can evoke this pattern of maladjustment.

Common causes of child and adolescent trauma include physical and sexual abuse and maltreatment, community and domestic violence, natural disasters, war, and civil conflicts (Putnam, 1996). However, it appears clear from the available clinical and empirical literature that the various types of traumatic events just mentioned do not *inevitably* lead to Posttraumatic Stress Disorder (McNally, 1993). These highly distressing experiences may be sufficient to elicit Posttraumatic Stress Disorder, but they are neither necessary nor inexorably sufficient. In the current social climate, it may be worth emphasizing that this is as true of sexual victimization (rape, incest, or other acute or chronic forms of sexual abuse) as of other types of traumatic events; the tendency at present is to assume that sexual abuse invariably results in Posttraumatic Stress Disorder, but this is not the case. The topics of risk factors and of possible protective factors (both subject variables and posttrauma experiences) are very exciting points of investigation in this area. Suffice it to say here that automatically diagnosing Posttraumatic Stress Disorder for any child with a history of sexual abuse (or any other traumatic experience) would lead to many errors of classification and constitute a misuse of this category, as supported by a 59-study meta-analysis (Rind, Tromovitch, & Bauserman, 1998).

The Defining Symptom Pattern

As noted earlier, the essential symptom picture for Posttraumatic Stress Disorder involves the manifestation of three (in children 6 years old and under) or all four (in those over age 6) elements: reexperiencing of the traumatic event; heightened arousal; and avoidance of stimuli connected with the trauma and/or changes in cognition and mood associated with the traumatic event(s). All of these symptoms must represent a change in the individual's typical behavior. Several specific symptom manifestations can be used to document each of these defining elements. All three or four, depending on age, must be present for the diagnosis to be made. In line with research examining the expression of Posttraumatic Stress Disorder in children (e.g., Scheeringa, Zeanah, & Cohen, 2011), a positive change in DSM-5 is the explicit presentation of alternative criteria for young children up to 6 years old. Blom and Oberink (2012) offer valuable discussions of the factor structure and developmental features of Posttraumatic Stress Disorder symptoms. The general statement of necessary functional impairment is included in the diagnostic criteria. The duration of troublesome symptoms must be at least 1 month.

The identified rate of Posttraumatic Stress Disorder is closely tied to the diagnostic criterion set used, and the changes from DSM-III to DSM-III-R to DSM-IV have had significant effects on the population of children classified with this disorder (Schwarz & Kowalski, 1991). Given this history, it is likely that the rate of Posttraumatic Stress Disorder diagnosis will change again with the application of the new DSM-5 criteria. Schwarz and Kowalski (1991) have also commented on the effects of different assessment methodologies (a self-report questionnaire for adults vs. structured interviews for children) on the detection of Posttraumatic Stress Disorder symptoms following a traumatic event. Serial assessment of children exposed to a trauma who show subsyndromal symptoms may be helpful in giving the examiner more opportunity to directly observe possible manifestations of avoidance, arousal, or reexperiencing phenomena. Although DSM-5 offers a new separate set of criteria for children 6 years of age and younger, this recommendation for repeated assessment is particularly relevant to very young children whose diagnoses are complicated by their developmental status.

Motta (1995) provides a nice review of Posttraumatic Stress Disorder for school psychologists, including a discussion of frequently observed and reported manifestations in a school setting and a review of assessment instruments and structured interviews. Motta appropriately comments that although such instruments can be helpful in eliciting data supporting a diagnosis of Posttraumatic Stress Disorder, assessment results are not the definitive standard: "Rather, school mental health personnel often make judgments based on multiple sources of input including data obtained from actual child behavior, oral report, test and questionnaire data, and the reports of those familiar with the child" (1995, p. 70). This statement is very consistent with the philosophy and clinical application of DSM-5. Fitzgerald and Cohen (2012) provide a useful summary of symptoms that may be manifested at school by children experiencing Posttraumatic Stress Disorder. They also provide a summary of efficacious cognitive-behavioral treatments for Posttraumatic Stress Disorder in the schools.

Epidemiological studies have found Posttraumatic Stress Disorder disturbingly frequent in youth. McLaughlin and colleagues (2013) found that 61.8% of adolescents had been exposed to a potentially traumatic experience, and they estimated a lifetime prevalence of Posttraumatic Stress Disorder of 4.7% based on DSM-IV-TR criteria. Giaconia and colleagues (1995) found that by age 18 more than 6% of a community sample of young people had met criteria for a diagnosis of Posttraumatic Stress Disorder at some point in their lives. They also found that partial symptomatology was common and could be very disabling even when full criteria for the diagnosis were not met. Pfefferbaum's (1997) review recommended clinical consideration of partial syndromes for treatment, especially in children for whom the chronic course of untreated Posttraumatic Stress Disorder can disrupt development.

The Course of Posttraumatic Stress Disorder

DSM-5 notes that Posttraumatic Stress Disorder can occur at any age and that the symptom picture may fluctuate over time. Complete recovery is reported to occur in roughly half of clinical cases within 3 months (p. 277); however, some cases persist stubbornly over many years. A troublesome issue in clinical practice is that as the symptom picture improves, either over time or in response to effective treatment, a child may no longer fully meet the criteria for Posttraumatic Stress Disorder. This can initially be dealt with by describing the disorder as In Partial Remission, but as the child continues to improve, a decision regarding reclassification will eventually be necessary. DSM-5 does not offer any guidance here. Our own practice is to view the reexperiencing of the trauma as the unique core of this diagnosis and to maintain the diagnosis as long as it is evident in the clinical picture.

Avoidance and overarousal are features of several Anxiety Disorders and are not unique to Posttraumatic Stress Disorder; thus the continuation of only these symptoms is not sufficient to retain this diagnostic formulation.

Significant comorbidities are reported for other Anxiety Disorders, as well as for Major Depressive Disorder, Bipolar Disorder, Conduct Disorder, and Substance-Related Disorders. In young children, Oppositional Defiant Disorder and Separation Anxiety Disorder are often seen accompanying Posttraumatic Stress Disorder diagnoses. Most clinical cases of Posttraumatic Stress Disorder meet criteria for another mental disorder. Substance involvement (alcohol use, as well as illicit and prescription drug use) should be carefully reviewed, especially in chronic cases. Deykin and Buka (1997) found gender differences in patterns of comorbidity between Substance Dependence and Posttraumatic Stress Disorder. The female adolescents in this study tended to develop chemical dependency after the establishment of Posttraumatic Stress Disorder, possibly to control the emotional distress associated with the stress reaction. In the male adolescents, the Substance Dependence tended to be the primary disorder that in turn led to Posttraumatic Stress Disorder by causing the teenagers to be exposed to situations in which traumatization was more likely.

Acute Stress Disorder

The diagnostic category of Acute Stress Disorder refers to the development of characteristic anxiety and dissociative symptoms within the first month following exposure to a traumatic event qualifying as sufficient for Posttraumatic Stress Disorder; the duration (the defining feature) is more than 3 days and less than 1 month. The symptom picture is identical to that of Posttraumatic Stress Disorder, with one major exception: The duration is restricted, as just noted. The disorder must develop more than 3 days, but no more than 1 month, after exposure to the traumatic event and last no more than 1 month. If maladjustment persists beyond a month, the diagnosis should be changed to another mental disorder (possibly Posttraumatic Stress Disorder, possibly some other mental disorder or syndrome).

Acute Stress Disorder and Posttraumatic Stress Disorder are mutually exclusive because of the duration elements in the definitions. The addition of a diagnosis of Posttraumatic Stress Disorder is a redefinition of the same symptom picture that has been used to document Acute Stress Disorder. The two disorders should not be concurrently diagnosed.

Importantly, DSM-5, unlike its predecessor, does not require the presence of dissociative symptoms for a diagnosis of Acute Stress Disorder. Dissociative symptoms are common in individuals who have lived through traumatic events, regardless of whether they subsequently develop Acute Stress Disorder or Posttraumatic Stress Disorder. Assessment of dissociative symptoms can be problematic. Scales assessing dissociative experiences have been developed for use with children (Putnam, Helmers, & Trickett, 1993) and adolescents (Armstrong, Putnam, Carlson, Libero, & Smith, 1997), and these can be of help in evaluating these symptom areas. (See also "Dissociation Disorders," Chapter 10, this volume.)

It is worth reiterating that neither sexual abuse nor any other traumatic event is necessarily sufficient to elicit the symptoms of Posttraumatic Stress Disorder, nor by extension do they guarantee development of Acute Stress Disorder. Exposure to an extremely traumatic experience is necessary for these two diagnoses but it is not sufficient; the diagnoses require the subsequent development of a characteristic symptom pattern.

Adjustment Disorders

Anxiety symptoms can also occur as a reaction to situational stressors in an individual's life. The diagnosis of Adjustment Disorder With Anxiety identifies the development of anxiety symptoms that cause distress or functional impairment (criteria for a mental disorder) and that develop following an identified psychosocial stressor. (Two other subtypes of Adjustment Disorder that involve, or can involve, anxiety symptoms—Adjustment Disorder With Mixed Anxiety and Depressed Mood and Adjustment Disorder With Mixed Disturbance of Emotions and Conduct—are mentioned in the previous chapter.) The relation of Adjustment Disorders to other disorders is structured by several rules that constrain the use of this diagnostic group. An Adjustment Disorder diagnosis is not made if the problems focused on can be accounted for by another Mental Disorder, even when this disorder appears clearly related etiologically to a psychosocial stressor. For instance, suppose that in apparent response to a bad experience in speaking before his class, a school-age boy shows over the next 6 months a recurrent and persistent fear of public speaking in all situations; responds to required class presentations with evidence of tremor, crying, sweating, and complaints of choking, nausea, and dizziness; attempts to avoid public speaking at almost any cost; and, because of this avoidance, passes up a chance to run for a position as class officer (which he has previously expressed interest in) and reports dreading school (which he has previously enjoyed). The diagnosis in this case should be Social Anxiety Disorder, Performance Only. This child meets all the criteria for Social Anxiety Disorder, and therefore this diagnosis is made rather than the diagnosis of Adjustment Disorder With Anxiety.

A diagnosis of Adjustment Disorder is also not made if the problem is seen as a stress-induced exacerbation of an existing disorder. For instance, if a girl who has previously met criteria for Social Anxiety Disorder, Performance Only (because of performance anxiety in social situations that caused her clinically significant distress) now begins to manifest active avoidance behavior of group events and parties because she has suffered extreme embarrassment at a social function, the diagnosis of Adjustment Disorder should not be added. The additional symptoms appear to be a further development of the Social Anxiety Disorder already present.

Furthermore, a diagnosis of Adjustment Disorder is not made if the symptoms persist more than 6 months after the termination of the stressor or its consequences. DSM-5 allows greater flexibility in recognizing that stressors may continue to influence functioning longer than 6 months and an Adjustment Disorder diagnosis can retained, but there is still a requirement of a temporal relation between the stressor and the disordered behavior. Previous editions placed rigid time limits on the use of Adjustment Disorder, a constriction that ignored not-uncommon real-life circumstances: Stressors are sometimes chronic (e.g., a parent's lingering illness) or create problems that persist over time (e.g., financial and interpersonal disruption caused by a parent's job loss). Shifting the criterion from the absolute duration of the disorder to the duration relative to the stressor means that these cases can be more sensibly handled. Adjustment Disorders, however, are viewed as essentially transient events that should eventually resolve. Persistence of the symptoms 6 months beyond the termination of the stressful precipitating events or their consequences requires a change of the diagnosis to another category—often Other Specified or Unspecified diagnosis within the general problem area.

The question of choosing between Adjustment Disorder With Anxiety and Other Specified or Unspecified Anxiety Disorder can be problematic for the examiner and is not completely resolved by DSM-5. These diagnoses should not be made if a child's or adolescent's symptom picture fully meets the criteria for any specific Anxiety Disorder diagnosis. The diagnosis of Adjustment Disorder should be made if there is evidence of anxiety symptoms (as the primary problems) that emerged within 3 months of the onset of an identifiable stressor, were in clear response to that stressor, and have not persisted for more than 6 months. The diagnosis of Other Specified or Unspecified Anxiety Disorder should be made if there is evidence of anxiety symptoms (as the primary problems) that have not been clearly precipitated by an identifiable situational event. The diagnosis of Other Specified or Unspecified Anxiety Disorder should also be made if the problems have persisted for more than 6 months after the resolution of the stressors and/or their consequences. Problematic cases involve symptoms lasting up to 6 months whose relation to events in the young person's life is questionable. The clear intention of DSM-5 (similar to previous editions) appears to be to constrain the use of Adjustment Disorder diagnoses to a set of distinct circumstances. Adjustment Disorder was one of the DSM-III-R diagnoses most frequently used with children and adolescents (Newcorn & Strain,

1992), and there has continued to be concern about the potential overuse of this category. Our recommendation is to use an Other Specified or Unspecified diagnosis if there is any real question regarding the identification of a stress-related disturbance linked to the difficulties with anxiety.

COMORBIDITY

A good heuristic rule to keep in mind with respect to Anxiety Disorders is that comorbidity tends to be the rule rather than the exception (Rapee, Schniering, & Hudson, 2009). Comorbid diagnoses of depressive disorders, Attention-Deficit/Hyperactivity Disorder, and other Anxiety Disorders are common. The frequently reported high correlations between specific Anxiety Disorders raise serious questions about the ultimate utility and validity of the DSM-5 approach to categorizing anxiety problems. The practical implications are that evidence of an Anxiety Disorder in a child or adolescent should prompt a careful review for possible evidence of other Anxiety Disorders, as well as a review of symptoms of Mood Disorders and Attention-Deficit/Hyperactivity Disorder. In adolescents, a careful evaluation of alcohol and other substance use should also be made.

CHILD MALTREATMENT

Child abuse and neglect in all manifestations are horrible breakdowns of caretaking that blight the lives of too many children. Despite increased public and professional concern and recognition of these topics over the past decades, it remains a challenge to obtain trustworthy prevalence estimates. Issues of definition, securing veridical reporting, and obtaining representative samples complicate our continuing efforts to monitor the incidence of pathological care of youth. Neglect and psychological abuse may well be more common than the more blatant cases of physical and sexual abuse that, in some instances at least, are easier to detect. Whatever the actual incidence is, it is too high. The sequelae of neglect and abuse are all too evident in the lives of many clients seen in the mental health systems. Abuse and neglect continue to be pressing social concerns in our nation.

Despite their deleterious effects, child abuse or neglect, no matter how extreme, are not Mental Disorders. Again, Mental Disorders are patterns of symptoms produced by an individual. The results of abusive treatment could well be Mental Disorders (e.g., Posttraumatic Stress Disorder, Acute Stress Disorder, Adjustment Disorder, Reactive Attachment Disorder, Disinhibited Social Engagement Disorder), but the act itself is not. In DSM-5, child abuse and neglect are included in the chapter "Other Conditions That

May Be a Focus of Clinical Attention." This chapter covers a variety of important categories that may well require intervention but that do not fall within the DSM-5 definition of a Mental Disorder. DSM-5 provides a much-expanded list of diagnostic codes from ICD-9-CM/ICD-10 for identification of child physical, sexual, and/or psychological abuse and child neglect. Separate codes are provided depending on whether the focus of clinical attention is on the victim or the perpetrator of the abuse or neglect, whether the contact is initial or subsequent, and whether the encounter is for mental health services.

10

Other Internalizing Problems

OVERVIEW

Several remaining groups of problems fall within the empirical cluster usually identified as "internalizing" or "overcontrolled" patterns. These include concerns and problems with a physical focus but without apparent medical basis, complaints that are primarily motivated by psychological needs, and disturbances in the integrity of the sense of self or other executive functions. In general, these disturbances in children and adolescents have received less empirical study than the other internalizing disorders, and less is known with confidence about them. To some extent, this difference reflects their lower base rate among clinical (and presumably the general) child and adolescent populations; however, it also reflects a greater lack of basic consensus among investigators and practitioners about the nature and even the reality of these phenomena in youth.

SOMATIC SYMPTOM AND RELATED DISORDERS

Somatic Symptom and Related Disorders present with physical symptoms or concerns that are not completely explained by general medical conditions. Importantly, disorders in this category are grouped together because of the presence of positive symptoms—that is, distressing somatic concerns coupled with abnormal thoughts, feelings, and behavior—rather than the absence of a medical diagnosis. Disorders in this category are more often seen in medical settings than in mental health or school settings. With these disorders, there is no indication that clients are deliberately faking, lying, or misrepresenting their experience, with the notable exception of Factitious Disorder. Clients with Somatic Symptom and Related Disorders appear to be sincerely experiencing the difficulties they are reporting to their physicians, but a full understanding of their problems usually cannot be achieved on the basis of the demonstrable physical findings. The DSM-5 chapter on Somatic Symptom and Related Disorders includes Psychological Factors Affecting Other Medical Conditions (see later in the chapter), in which there is a medical condition that can be diagnosed.

It is difficult to state with any confidence how common these phenomena may be, especially in children and adolescents. A general recommendation is for evaluators to be conservative with respect to Somatic Symptom and Related Disorder diagnoses. The consequences of missing a general medical condition may be much more serious than the consequences of delaying acceptance of a Somatic Symptom Disorder diagnosis. At a minimum, a Somatic Symptom Disorder diagnosis should be a positive diagnosis; that is, it should be "ruled in" by the available data. Such a diagnosis should not be made solely on the basis of there being no readily apparent biological basis for the problems; there must also be positive evidence that psychological factors play a significant role in the difficulties. Mrazek (1994) has reviewed difficulties in basing diagnoses on the absence of physical explanations for symptoms.

Examiners would also do well to remember that there is nothing about manifesting a Somatic Symptom (or Related) Disorder that ensures good physical health thereafter. When a child or adolescent has a well-documented Somatic Symptom Disorder, it is necessary to monitor his or her health carefully because caretakers are likely to assume that any new ache, pain, or limitation reported is another expression of the Mental Disorder. A distressingly high percentage of children diagnosed with Conversion Disorder, for example, have been found to have had a physical disorder that could account for their symptoms (Lehmkuhl, Blanz, Lehmkuhl, & Braum-Scharm, 1989). This finding is consistent with the adult literature, which reveals many patients diagnosed with Conversion Disorders to be eventually diagnosed with neurological disorders (Katon, 1993).

In a review of research in this area, Fritz, Fritsch, and Hagino (1997) point out that progress was hampered by diagnostic criteria that were developed for adults and are often not useful for children and adolescents. Preliminary evidence suggests that the advent of new diagnostic categories for somatic symptoms is a welcome addition for diagnosis of youth (Schulte & Petermann, 2011). These authors found that the diagnostic criteria for Somatic Symptom Disorder are more appropriate for classifying children and adolescents relative to the old diagnostic criteria for DSM-IV

Somatoform Disorders. Only time will tell whether these changes lead to better outcomes, but it is clear that this area is in great need of further study and development. The next IDEA Note addresses how Somatic Symptom and Related Disorders may lead to eligibility for special education services under IDEA. The DSM-IV note on pages 138–139 discusses changes made to this general diagnostic category in DSM-5 from the last version of DSM.

Somatic Symptom Disorder

Presentation of Somatic Symptom Disorder, a new disorder in DSM-5, involves the client reporting multiple somatic complaints and symptoms that cannot be demonstrated to have a physiological basis. Importantly, the disorder is diagnosed based on the presence of somatic complaints coupled with abnormal thoughts, feelings, and behavior that interfere with functioning. This conceptualization is a departure from the approach to Somatoform Disorders covered in DSM-IV-TR in that the focus has shifted away from the absence of a medical diagnosis to the presence of psychological symptoms. The influence of this shift is still unknown, particularly for children and adolescents. According to DSM-5, the criteria for this disorder capture approximately 75% of clients who would have previously met the

IDEA Note. Somatic Symptom and Related Disorders and IDEA

A diagnosis of a Somatic Symptom and Related Disorder can form the basis for qualifying a child for special education services under the "serious emotional disturbance" category of IDEA. One of the identified conditions indicating a serious emotional disturbance is a "tendency to develop physical symptoms or fears associated with personal or school problems" that persists "over a period of time" and "adversely affects educational performance" (Individuals with Disabilities Education Improvement Act, 2004; Public Law 108-446, paragraph (c)(4)(i)). Severe somatic symptoms fall within this condition. Another identified condition is "an inability to build or maintain satisfactory relationships with peers and teachers," which can be a consequence of Somatic Symptom and Related Disorders in children and adolescents. Documentation of the functional impairment caused by the Somatic Symptom and Related Disorder on academic or social adjustment will be important. Information regarding the psychosocial and environmental influences and the child's overall functioning may also be important in establishing eligibility for services under IDEA. As previously discussed for anxiety and mood problems (see the IDEA Notes on pp. 86 and 110–111, it is necessary under IDEA to document the effect of an emotional disturbance on educational performance.

criteria for the now-defunct diagnosis of Hypochondriasis. Illness Anxiety Disorder was developed to capture the remaining 25% who do not have remarkable somatic symptoms but do evince strong fears about their health that interfere with functioning.

Somatic Symptom and Related Disorders are historically diagnosed in adults, but the behaviors may have begun in adolescence or childhood. Fritz and colleagues (1997) suggest that the infrequency of diagnosis in youth is the result of developmentally inappropriate criteria rather than the absence of the phenomenon. The literature on childhood depression suggests that young children often express emotional distress in terms of physical complaints. Nonspecific abdominal pain and headaches are relatively frequent somatic symptoms in youth (Fritz et al., 1997). It is hoped that continued investigation will contribute more developmentally useful formulations of somatic behavior in young people.

Illness Anxiety Disorder

The new diagnosis of Illness Anxiety Disorder captures approximately a quarter of cases that were formerly diagnosed as Hypochondriasis who do not qualify for a diagnosis of Somatic Symptom Disorder. In contrast with those diagnosed with Somatic Symptom Disorder, clients experiencing Illness Anxiety Disorder report no (or only minor) somatic symptoms, but they report extreme worry about their medical well-being that interferes with their functioning. It is manifested in fears of and preoccupations with being unwell. The authors of DSM-5 acknowledge Illness Anxiety Disorder as an Anxiety Disorder but positioned it in the "Somatic Symptom and Related Disorders" chapter because it almost exclusively presents within a medical setting as opposed to a mental health or school setting.

In our experience, children and adolescents who demonstrate frequent concerns about health in the absence of a history of critical health problems often have a family pattern of high sensitivity to possible illness and symptoms of illness. There may be a family history of a critical, debilitating, or fatal illness in a sibling or a child from a previous generation. A critical intervention goal is to help the young person and family avoid extinguishing appropriate adult concern to reports of potentially important physical symptoms.

Conversion Disorder

Conversion Disorder is characterized by the appearance of a problem with motor control or sensory functioning that would usually suggest a neurological or other medical problem but is without demonstrable biological foundation. The symptom pattern is usually focused and relatively stable, in contrast to the many and fluctuating symptoms of Somatic Symptom Disorder. Conversion Disorder is subclassified in terms of type of symptom or deficit (i.e., With Weakness or Paralysis, With Abnormal Movement, With Swallowing Symptoms, With Speech Symptoms, With Attacks or Seizures, With Anesthesia or Sensory Loss, With Special Sensory Symptom, or With Mixed Symptoms), by duration of symptoms (Acute Episode or Persistent), and by presence of an identified stressor (With Psychological Stressor or Without Psychological Stressor).

Although case studies of Conversion Disorder have been the basis for much theoretical discussion, empirical studies are infrequent. Siegel and Barthel (1986) reported on the frequency of several characteristics of Conversion Disorder in a pediatric sample. They found evidence of an identifiable psychosocial stress in 89% of these cases, a model for conversion symptoms in 56%, and family dysfunction in 56%. There was evidence of secondary gain in 41% of these cases. In a more recent study of 240 childhood cases of Conversion Disorder, Ani, Reading, Lynn, Forlee, and Garralda (2013) found that motor weaknesses, abnormal movements, and pseudoseizures are the conversion symptoms most frequently reported in children. Classic Conversion Disorder, involving paralysis or loss of sensory functions (e.g., "hysterical paralysis" of the legs or "hysterical blindness"), seems relatively rare today in adults but continues to be seen occasionally in children. Conversion Disorder involving neurological phenomena ("pseudoseizures") may be more common.

The diagnostic dilemma in child neurological cases may be great because of the reported occurrence both of seizures with a clear neurological basis and of pseudoseizures in the same children. Both careful evaluation and skillful intervention are required to manage and treat these children effectively. Wynick, Hobson, and Jones (1997) report that cases of psychogenic disorders of vision, or "visual conversion reactions," are often seen by ophthalmologists rather than mental health professionals; such cases tend to be related to environmental stress and respond well to suggestion or reassurance.

In our clinical experiences, Conversion Disorder in children and adolescents has usually been associated with significant family conflict and with inconsistency both in expectations for the youth and in consequences for behavior. There is often a precipitating stressor for the original manifestation of the problem, but this stressor cannot always be identified with certainty. The waxing and waning of symptoms are usually associated with increased and decreased psychological stress within the young persons' family, school, and/or community experience. Associations with other somatic symptoms and occasionally other Somatic Symptom and Related Disorders occur. Associations with dependent and oppositional personality traits can sometimes be seen. Comorbid or possible future diagnoses of Anxiety

Disorders (especially Panic Disorder), Depressive Disorders, Somatic Symptom Disorder, and neurological and other medical conditions should be considered and ruled in or out. DSM-5 suggests a higher co-occurrence with Personality Disorders than in the general population; however, even if this is the case, these diagnoses usually cannot be made with confidence in a child or adolescent (Antisocial Personality Disorder cannot be diagnosed prior to age 18).

Both high suggestibility and secondary gain (positive or negative reinforcement, usually unintentional, of sick role behavior) are commonly found in children and adolescents with Conversion Disorder, but these characteristics have a high base rate in the general population and in clinical populations. We do not think that suggestibility or evidence of secondary gain can be used with any confidence to rule in Conversion Disorder. Similarly, an apparent lack of concern over symptoms (*la belle indifference*) can be an associated feature of Conversion Disorder, but it too lacks adequate positive or negative predictive value to be accorded significant diagnostic weight. Siegel and Barthel (1986) found evidence of secondary gain in 41% of their cases and *la belle indifference* in 30%.

Psychological Factors Affecting Other Medical Conditions

Psychological Factors Affecting Other Medical Conditions was upgraded to a Mental Disorder in DSM-5. This category is used to identify cases in which there are extant medical or physical problems in an individual's life and also evidence that psychological factors play a significant role in the exacerbation or maintenance of these medical difficulties. The role of good clinical judgment is especially important with this category. Psychological factors probably play a role in most disease and recovery courses, but this category is intended to note those instances in which the role is of marked importance in understanding cases and managing them effectively. Close cooperation and frequent communication between the medical professionals involved and the school psychologist constitute the best basis for both identifying and responding helpfully to these cases.

Other Specified Somatic Symptom and Related Disorder and Unspecified Somatic Symptom and Related Disorder

Other Specified Somatic Symptom and Related Disorder and Unspecified Somatic Symptom and Related Disorder are residual diagnostic categories for cases of Somatic Symptom and Related Disorders that do not fully meet the criteria for identified patterns. For example, Pseudocyesis (a mistaken belief that one is pregnant, associated with some of the usual objective signs of pregnancy) is occasionally seen in adolescent females; such cases are diagnosed as Other Specified Somatic Symptom and Related Disorder. A diagnosis of Unspecified Somatic Symptom and Related Disorder was intended to be given rarely when inadequate information is available to provide a more definitive diagnosis.

Factitious Disorder

Factitious Disorder reflects the deliberate feigning of symptoms of a Mental Disorder or General Medical Condition, with the only apparent motivation being that of assuming the role of patient. In contrast with Malingering (discussed later), there is an absence of clear external reinforcement (payoff) for the sick role. The few times either of us has seen this behavior in adolescents, it was always associated with other Mental Disorders. Factitious Disorder differs from the other disorders in the "Somatic Symptom and Related Disorders" chapter of DSM-5 in that the problems and complaints are intentionally and knowingly concocted. That is, individuals with Factitious Disorder (like those exhibiting Malingering) are aware of "putting on."

Factitious Disorder Imposed on Another is a special case of Factitious Disorder. These include cases in which the deception involves one person claiming and/or producing symptoms in another (usually a parent provoking unnecessary medical attention for a child)—"factitious disorder by proxy." Similar to other cases of Factitious Disorder, the goal of the perpetrator is solely to gain status or attention for the sick role of the victim.

DSM-IV Note. Changes in DSM-5 for Somatic Symptom and Related Disorders

Several major changes were made to the class of disorders covered in the DSM-5 "Somatic Symptom and Related Disorders" chapter. Four disorders were removed (i.e., Somatization Disorder, Undifferentiated Somatoform Disorder, Pain Disorder, and Hypochondriasis). Body Dysmorphic Disorder, formerly covered in the Somatoform Disorders chapter of DSM-IV-TR, appears in the "Obsessive–Compulsive and Related Disorders" chapter of DSM-5. Two new disorders were added, namely Somatic Symptom Disorder and Illness Anxiety Disorder. One disorder—Conversion Disorder—remains with only modest changes. Factitious Disorder, covered in a freestanding chapter in DSM-IV-TR, and Psychological Factors Affecting Other Medical Conditions, covered in the "Other Conditions That May Be a Focus of Clinical Attention" chapter in DSM-IV-TR, are included in the "Somatic Symptom and Related Disorders" chapter of DSM-5. Somatoform Disorder Not Otherwise Specified was replaced with Other Specified and Unspecified Somatic Symptom and Related Disorder categories. Thus, the seven disorders in the "Somatic Symptom and Related Disorders" chapter are: Somatic

Symptom Disorder, Illness Anxiety Disorder, Conversion Disorder (Functional Neurological Symptom Disorder), Psychological Factors Affecting Other Medical Conditions, Factitious Disorder, Other Specified Somatic Symptom and Related Disorder, and Unspecified Somatic Symptom and Related Disorder. The changes made to the diagnostic criteria for the three disorders in this chapter with similar coverage in DSM-IV-TR are detailed here.

Conversion Disorder (Functional Neurological Symptom Disorder)

DSM-5 criteria for Conversion Disorder are less stringent than they were in DSM-IV-TR. The criteria no longer require that stressors precede the symptoms or deficit. It also no longer includes the criterion that the symptom is not intentionally produced or feigned. The specifiers are more detailed in terms of symptom type and duration relative to those provided in DSM-IV-TR.

Psychological Factors Affecting Other Medical Conditions

The specifiers for this disorder were reduced to cover only severity, not the source of psychological factors thought to explain the disturbance and the influenced medical condition.

Factitious Disorder

DSM-5 does not include the criterion that the person's motivation is to assume the sick role, as required by DSM-IV-TR. Factitious Disorder in DSM-5 includes specifiers for frequency (i.e., Single Episode or Recurrent Episodes) and the target (i.e., Factitious Disorder Imposed on Self vs. Factitious Disorder Imposed on Another, which was previously known as Factitious Disorder by Proxy).

OTHER MENTAL DISORDERS/CONDITIONS INVOLVING PRESENTATION OF PHYSICAL SYMPTOMS

Nonadherence to Medical Treatment

Nonadherence to Medical Treatment is one of the Other Conditions That May Be a Focus of Clinical Attention (not a Mental Disorder in DSM-5), applicable to situations in which clinical attention needs to be focused on the client's failure to cooperate with treatment. This noncompliance can be associated with normal child or adolescent development, with other situations that are best conceptualized in terms of V codes (e.g., Parent–Child Relational Problem), or with a specific Mental Disorder (e.g., Oppositional Defiant Disorder). Regardless of the context, the matter is serious enough to warrant clinical attention and hence formal identification. The potential effects can range from minor annoyances to life-threatening medical consequences (e.g., a boy with diabetes who refuses to control his alcohol intake; a girl with previously well-controlled phenylketonuria (PKU) who will not adhere to the dietary restrictions that make her stand out from her peer group).

Malingering

Malingering is the V code used to classify intentional "faking" of symptoms or a disorder in order to achieve some desired end. Distinguishing between Malingering and Factitious Disorder centers on external motivation, according to DSM-5. In cases of Malingering, there is a clear external incentive for feigning illness, such as monetary gain or being excused from work or military duty. In contrast, external motivators are not seen in cases of Factitious Disorder. It is the presence of an identifiable payoff or external incentive that differentiates Malingering from Factitious Disorder; it is the conscious, intentional aspect that differentiates Malingering from Conversion Disorder. A trivial manifestation in children and adolescents is feigning illness to avoid school for a day. Much more serious is feigning Attention-Deficit/Hyperactivity Disorder in order to obtain a prescription for a stimulant medication to be misused or resold.

Adjustment Disorder, Unspecified

Occasionally the psychologist will see physical complaints that have developed in response to psychosocial stress and appear to meet the general criteria of a Mental Disorder. These can be diagnosed as Adjustment Disorder, Unspecified.

DISSOCIATIVE DISORDERS

Dissociative Disorders all reflect a "disruption of and/or discontinuity in the normal integration of consciousness, memory, identity, emotion, perception, body representation, motor control, and behavior" (p. 291). Although dissociative symptoms are common in both typical development and many mental disorders, we advise caution in making a Dissociative Disorder diagnosis in children or adolescents, especially as a primary diagnosis. Great controversy surrounds this topic, and unfortunately "more heat than light" is currently being offered in much of the available literature on both sides of the controversy. The development of instruments such as the Child Dissociative Checklist, a parent report dissociative checklist (Putnam et al., 1993), and the Adolescent Dissociative Experiences Scale, an adolescent self-report measure (Armstrong et al., 1997), may help guide clinical evaluation in this area—as similar checklists have helped move the

IDEA Note. Dissociative Disorders and IDEA

Although dissociative experiences appear to be relatively common and unremarkable in children, severe and enduring dissociative phenomena that cause marked distress or impair social or academic adjustment (i.e., Dissociative Disorders) are rare among children and adolescents, in our experiences. If a severe Dissociative Disorder is diagnosed in a young person, it can probably serve as the basis for eligibility for special education services under IDEA through several of the conditions identifying "severe emotional disturbance." If dissociative symptoms interfere with learning, they can meet the criterion of "an inability to learn which cannot be explained by intellectual, sensory, or health factors." If dissociative symptoms interfere with social relationships, they can thus cause "an inability to build or maintain satisfactory relationships with peers and teachers." Finally, if dissociative symptoms lead to socially deviant actions or unusual emotional responses, they result in "inappropriate types of behavior or feelings under normal circumstances" (Individuals with Disabilities Education Improvement Act, 2004, Public Law 108-446, paragraph (c)(4)(i)). As previously discussed for anxiety and mood problems (see the two IDEA Notes on pp. 86 and 110–111, it is necessary under IDEA to document the effect of an emotional disturbance on educational performance.

assessment of attention deficits onto a more objective and empirically based foundation. The IDEA Note above sets forth how Dissociative Disorders relate to eligibility for special education services under IDEA.

Dissociative Amnesia

Dissociative Amnesia (Psychogenic Amnesia in DSM-III and DSM-III-R) refers to loss of important personal information that is too excessive for normal forgetting and not accounted for by another Dissociative Disorder, Posttraumatic Stress Disorder, Acute Stress Disorder, Somatic Symptom Disorder, or a Neurocognitive Disorder. Symptoms of dissociative amnesia occur in children and adolescents, often as part of the clinical picture of a trauma reaction. DSM-5 notes that differential diagnosis of Dissociative Amnesia in children is complicated by several developmental features, and multiple sources of data are often necessary (p. 299).

DSM-5 incorporates the former freestanding disorder Dissociative Fugue into the Dissociative Amnesia diagnostic criteria as a specifier. It indicates that the confusion about or amnesia for an individual's previous identity is accompanied by wandering or intentional travel. The problem is rare in general, and even more so in adolescents; onset is usually associated with traumatic events or overwhelming stress. Careful evaluation is needed to rule out Malingering, Psychotic Disorders, Manic Episodes, and neurological disorders with complex partial (temporal lobe or psychomotor) seizures.

Dissociative Identity Disorder

Dissociative Identity Disorder (known as Dissociative Identity Disorder in DSM-IV and DSM-IV-TR, Multiple Personality Disorder in DSM-III-R, and Multiple Personality in DSM-III) is still often referred to by the acronym MPD for Multiple Personality Disorder, the historical label for the phenomenon. A related concept is "false-memory syndrome," an expression used by those who challenge the validity of the frequent use of Dissociative Identity Disorder as an explanation for difficult-to-understand clinical cases. Clinicians who were uncomfortable with the idea of one body having more than one personality were more welcoming of the DSM-IV label change (that has been maintained in DSM-5), as it was easier to accept the idea of one body having more than one identity. There are more than semantic niceties involved here; issues of criminal responsibility, the validity of "recovered memories," the choice of acceptable therapeutic goals, and other critical concerns are at stake. This diagnostic category marks one set of limits about what we understand regarding the development and vicissitudes of a human's sense of self, identity, and personality. It is a small part of the answer to questions about when and under what circumstances a person should feel and be held accountable for the actions his or her body takes.

We generally recommend that diagnoses of Dissociative Identity Disorder in children or adolescents be made only after consultation with colleagues. To our knowledge, all major discussions in the literature note the frequent association of Dissociative Identity Disorder with Mood Disorders, Anxiety Disorders, Personality Disorders, Eating Disorders, Substance-Related Disorders, Sexual and Gender Identity Disorders, and occasionally Psychotic Disorders. In particular, comorbid diagnoses with Posttraumatic Stress Disorder, Substance-Related Disorders, Major Depressive Disorder, and Borderline Personality Disorder occur with some regularity. Although we are convinced that dissociative phenomena are real, the clinical utility of Dissociative Identity Disorder as a diagnostic category (rather than a therapeutic metaphor—an "as if you were") is not well established, particularly for use with children. Nevertheless, it is available as a diagnosis in DSM-5, and the phenomenon is reported in children and adolescents. Boyson (2011) provides a review of the literature on Dissociative Identity Disorder in children, noting minimal research on this rare disorder in this population.

Child battering, sexual exploitation and abuse, and/or neglect of basic developmental needs are common problems of pathological parenting reported to be associated with Dissociative Identity Disorder. DSM-5 includes the following three problems in the "Other Conditions That May Be a Focus of Clinical Attention" chapter: Child Physical Abuse, Child Sexual Abuse, and Child Neglect. Within this broad category, DSM-5 provides more specific classification regarding the type of encounter (initial vs. subsequent), status of the report (confirmed vs. suspected), and other circumstances related to the event (encounter with mental health services for victim of parental abuse vs. nonparental abuse, personal history of past abuse, and encounter of mental health services for perpetrator of parental vs. nonparental abuse). We discuss these conditions further in Chapter 9 of this book in reference to Anxiety Disorders.

Depersonalization/Derealization Disorder

As its names indicates, Depersonalization Disorder involves episodes of depersonalization—feelings of detachment or unreality regarding one's self—of Derealization—feelings of detachment and unreality regarding one's surroundings—or both. Occasional feelings of depersonalization and/or derealization are common both in normal adolescents and in adolescents with a wide variety of mental disorders. A diagnosis of Depersonalization Disorder is only made if the symptoms are frequent and intense enough to cause significant distress and/or impairment (i.e., they constitute a Mental Disorder) *and* if they occur independently of another Mental Disorder and the use of substances.

Other Specified and Unspecified Dissociative Disorder

The categories of Other Specified Dissociative Disorder and Unspecified Dissociative Disorder are used to classify a variety of unusual case presentations, responses to chronic exposure to coercive persuasion (e.g., recruitment into cults), dissociative trance disorders (culture-bound phenomena), and atypical cases similar to Dissociative Identity Disorder. The following Professional Note describes a condition called "dissociative hallucinosis" that appears to fall into this category.

Professional Note. Dissociative Hallucinosis

Nurcombe and colleagues (1996) discuss a condition they refer to as "dissociative hallucinosis," which appears to be a state with characteristics of Dissociative Disorders, Psychotic Disorders, and Posttraumatic Stress Disorder. Nurcombe and colleagues believe that there is a consistent phenomenon underlying a number of historical terms in psychopathology: "hysterical psychosis, hysterical hallucinations, hysterical twilight state, hysterical delirium, hysterical trance, hysterical pseudopsychosis, hysterical pseudoschizophrenia, hysterical pseudodementia, hypnoid state, somnambulistic crisis, psychological automatism, transient psychotic episode, episodic dyscontrol, and dissociative psychosis" (p. 109). They identify defining features (p. 110):

1. Acute onset, brief duration, and a recurrent course, but no personality deterioration.
2. Trance-like episodes of altered consciousness.
3. Hyperarousal and negative emotions (fear, anger).
4. Impulsive aggression, destructiveness, suicidal behavior, or self-injurious behavior.
5. Auditory and/or visual hallucinations, intrusive mental images, and nightmares.
6. Disorganized thinking.

The reliability and diagnostic/therapeutic validity of such a category remain to be convincingly demonstrated. The most appropriate DSM-5 diagnosis would probably be Other Specified Dissociative Disorder. We recommend evaluating carefully to rule out (or in) Borderline Personality Disorder, which can show similar symptoms: transient psychotic episodes, including vivid hallucinations; acute confusion and disorientation; intense negative affect; self-injurious, aggressive, and destructive actions; and dissociative phenomena.

11

Problems with Conduct

OVERVIEW

Familiar to school psychologists is the finding that the most frequent basis for a mental health referral from teachers or parents is some pattern of rule-defiant behaviors (Shamsie & Hluchy, 1991). Doll's (1996) review of epidemiological studies found that behavioral disorders (Conduct Disorder, Oppositional Disorder or Oppositional Defiant Disorder, and Attention Deficit Disorder or Attention-Deficit/Hyperactivity Disorder) were the most frequently diagnosed psychiatric disorders in school-age children. Nearly two decades later, these diagnoses continue to draw significant clinical attention in school settings (Hess, Pejic, & Castejon, 2014). Various labels have been used in the psychological literature to describe children who disobey adults, act in violation of understood expectations within a setting, attack their peers, and disrupt the cooperation of others in play or work. At the turn of the 20th century, the term "conduct problems" began to be used with increasing frequency. Psychodynamic writers referred to "acting-out behavior." Empirical analyses of the covariations between "externalizing" behaviors appeared. Advocates of behavior modification tended to speak of "oppositional behavior." Increasing empirical evidence began to accumulate that such problems are persistent, often get worse instead of better over time, and predict multiple negative outcomes for a child. Further reports brought increasing awareness that these problems are often difficult to treat and that traditional interventions have limited usefulness. Eventually empirical confirmation became available for what clinicians had feared: These behavior problems are associated with other serious problems—substance misuse and adult personality disturbances. Disruptive behavior problems remain among the most challenging areas of service for psychologists and other child care professionals.

Disruptive behavior problems in school settings manifest themselves in repeated conflictual encounters with peers, teachers, and other school personnel. Children with these problems are the ones most frequently corrected or reprimanded for their public behavior. They are usually well known to the school secretary, the building service worker, the playground supervisor, and the bus driver. Disruptive behavior problems can be situational, but they more typically occur across all of a child's environments, especially those situations that call for self-control, cooperative behavior, turn taking, and restraint in movement and activity. These problems tend to be overt and obvious to the adults in each setting (although the behaviors may not be perceived as "mental health problems"). Moreover, there can be relatively good correspondence between the reports of children with disruptive behavior problems and the reports of adults regarding them (Cantwell et al., 1997). However, whether such children qualify for services under IDEA is far less obvious and is a matter of continuing debate (see the next two IDEA Notes).

IDEA Note. Disruptive Behavior Disorders and IDEA

The diagnostic categories of DSM-5 do not automatically correspond to the eligibility categories identified in IDEA. Even when identical labels are used, the precise definitions (or absence of definitions) often leave open serious questions regarding the equivalence of the behavior problems outlined in the two systems. Some Disruptive Behavior Disorders would seem to fall within the area identified in IDEA as "emotional disturbance," if the disruptive behavior is a manifestation of an underlying emotional issue. (For a separate discussion of Attention-Deficit/Hyperactivity Disorder and IDEA, see the IDEA Note on p. 163.) One major emphasis in IDEA is a focus on disability conditions that handicap a child in achieving academic or vocational success. The increased attention in DSM-5 to the functional impairment criteria in almost all diagnoses has obvious relevance here. Mental disorders with symptoms that directly interfere with academic achievement or social development will be easier to establish as relevant for IDEA classification.

The essential feature of Conduct Disorder consists of repeated major rule violations and acts against the basic rights of others. The symptoms and consequences of Conduct Disorder will make it more difficult to support a classification under the "emotional disturbance" description category of IDEA. In our opinion, a strong case can usually be made for Oppositional Defiant Disorder and for Intermittent Explosive Disorder, given the serious and chronic nature of these problems and their more direct connection to emotion regulation deficits; however, efforts to document the effects of these disorders on scholastic achievement will be necessary to carry this case forward. An important change in DSM-5 is that Conduct Disorder and Oppositional Defiant Disorder diagnoses can now be made concurrently. In our experience, many or most youth with Conduct Disorder also have oppositional/defiant characteristics (which was the basis of the previous exclusion of Oppositional Defiant Disorder in the context of Conduct Disorder). The DSM-5 formulation of Oppositional Defiant Disorder has added an emphasis on the underlying emotional disturbance, which could facilitate the inclusion of children showing both Conduct Disorder and Oppositional Defiant Disorder under the "emotional disturbance" provisions of IDEA.

What is most important for the reader to recognize is that the categories of IDEA and DSM-5 do not automatically translate into each other. The basic purpose, structure, and methods of the two systems are different, and the "mapping" of one upon the other is imperfect and open to differences of interpretation. Establishing an objective case for a mental disorder diagnosis will usually support and facilitate qualification of a student as eligible for services under IDEA, provided that the disorder is connected to significant academic and/or interpersonal issues.

In the case of disruptive behavior, one of the biggest challenges in determining eligibility is the requisite that the problematic behavior be a manifestation of an underlying emotional disturbance. Requirements for the assessment methods and results necessary to document the connection between overt behavior and underlying emotional functioning vary by state and even local standards, making it especially challenging for the practicing school psychologist to advocate for youth with Conduct Disorder to receive special education services under the category of emotional disturbance. School districts sometimes adopt policies and procedures to place students with disruptive behavior in alternative, behavior-disordered programs rather than in special education placements when it is not clear that the behavior is connected to an underlying emotional disturbance. Such youth are considered "socially maladjusted" and are excluded from eligibility for special education services. This situation places pressure on the practicing school psychologist who may see a youth as in need of educational, social, and mental health services. Cases of Oppositional Defiant Disorder and Intermittent Explosive Disorder may be easier to make given the new diagnostic criteria (see the DSM-IV-TR Note on p. 151).

Furthermore, the establishment of several classifications in DSM-5 that are not Mental Disorders (the V codes) can also serve as a basis for seeking special education services under IDEA. Psychiatric classification can help document intellectual, personal, and social problems that limit a young person's success in school and in the community; this documentation has the potential to open the door for eligibility under IDEA. (However, see the IDEA Note on p. 148 for cautions about IDEA eligibility in such cases.)

IDEA Note. Cautions about Disruptive Behavior Disorders and IDEA

Considerable confusion and disagreement have surrounded the inclusion of children with serious conduct problems under IDEA. The definition of "emotional disturbance" in IDEA contains an exclusion for children whose behavior is "socially maladjusted" but does not fall within the specific conditions defined as "seriously emotionally disturbed." Unfortunately, no definition of "socially maladjusted" is given, so it is not clear what has been excluded. The usual interpretation is that delinquent behavior in isolation does not qualify a child as eligible for special services unless that child also meets one or more of the conditions identified as "seriously emotionally disturbed." Of some importance is that the act clearly does not exclude children who are "socially maladjusted"; it only indicates that social maladjustment alone is insufficient to establish eligibility under IDEA. Even more unfortunately, some state policies have been written to use DSM diagnoses of Conduct Disorder or Oppositional Defiant Disorder for exclusion from qualification under IDEA. Such a position would appear to be counter to the intention of the act (Cline, 1990; Council for Children with Behavioral Disorders, 1987) and at odds with the populations often served by special education (McGinnis, 1986).

Several groups of DSM-5 diagnoses deal with oppositional, rule-defiant, and aggressive behavior. First (2014) gives differential diagnosis decision trees for behavior problems in a child or adolescent that allow practitioners to examine classes of disorders systematically, although even his useful discussion omits some of the diagnoses that would have to be considered (e.g., Intermittent Explosive Disorder). Along with establishing the clearest diagnostic classification of a child's or adolescent's presenting concerns, the examiner should carefully consider any associated behavior problems the youth may be experiencing. Disruptive behavior problems tend to have high comorbidities with other psychiatric problems. As always, the general issue is how to "capture" all relevant clinical information about a young person and his or her problems and situation most effectively and efficiently. Among the frequently reported comorbid conditions for many of the disruptive problems are Depressive Disorders, Anxiety Disorders, Learning Disorders, Elimination Disorders, Communication Disorders, and Substance Use Disorders (usually in adolescence).

In addition to formal diagnoses, other pertinent individual differences can be recorded within the framework of DSM-5. Two such characteristics of relevance to disruptive behavior problems are early temperament and intelligence. The potential importance of early temperamental differences among children in the development of behavior problems is increasingly being recognized. As we noted in Chapter 3 in this volume, noncategorical information regarding personality traits and other characterological differences may be provided in the description leading up to a formal DSM-5 diagnosis. A child's intelligence is another variable that appears to interact with a history of behavior problems to affect prognosis; in general, higher intelligence appears to be associated with a better prognosis for later successful adjustment in children with such problems. Data about intellectual ability can also be noted in this description, even if it does not involve a diagnostic classification.

A childhood history of disruptive behavior problems has been associated with a number of serious adult diagnoses, notably Antisocial Personality Disorder, Borderline Personality Disorder, and Schizophrenia. Moreover, disruptive children are at high risk of social adjustment problems in adulthood even when they do not qualify for mental health diagnoses: Marital conflict, child abuse, occupational maladjustment, and legal problems are overrepresented in their follow-up evaluations. In general, it is not safe to assume that these children will outgrow their problems in adjusting to the expectations of others and of society.

Finally, a number of pathological environmental circumstances are overrepresented in the lives of many youth with disruptive behavior problems. The examiner should be alert to the presence in a youth's environment of abuse, neglect, and/or modeling of antisocial attitudes and behavior. A family history of criminal behavior, substance abuse, or mood disorders may contribute to the environmental adversity often seen in the backgrounds of these children.

DIFFERENTIAL DIAGNOSIS

One major pattern of behavior disturbance is a chronic history of serious rule violations; this behavior disturbance is the basic concept of a "conduct disorder" as the phrase is generally used in the psychological literature. Although some authors have questioned the validity of Conduct Disorder as a useful diagnosis (Lewis, Lewis, Unger, & Goldman, 1984), in general it is one of the best supported DSM diagnoses in both the empirical and clinical literature (Robins, 1991). In contrast, a habitual pattern of emotional dysregulation, defiant behavior, and vindictiveness that stops short of major rule violations or aggression against people or property is the essential feature of Oppositional Defiant Disorder. Conduct problems that do not meet criteria for Conduct Disorder and/or Oppositional Defiant Disorder and that appear in response to an identified stress may meet the criteria for Adjustment Disorder With Disturbance of Conduct. Intermittent Explosive Disorder is a pattern of repeated impulsive, aggressive behavior most commonly seen in children and adolescents. Bipolar I Disorder, Most

Recent Episode Manic is rare in children and infrequent in adolescents, but it does occur and may present with conduct symptoms. Finally, isolated acts of delinquent or antisocial behavior that do not constitute a pattern of maladjustment can be classified with the Child or Adolescent Antisocial Behavior detailed in the "Other Conditions That May Be a Focus of Clinical Attention" chapter (although this coding is not a Mental Disorder). Frequently associated diagnoses or problems that should be considered and ruled in or out when a child presents with apparent Conduct Disorder, Oppositional Defiant Disorder, Intermittent Explosive Disorder, or Other Specified or Unspecified Disruptive, Impulse-Control, and Conduct Disorder include Attention-Deficit/Hyperactivity Disorder, Substance Use Disorders, Learning Disorders, Mental Retardation, Mood Disorders, Anxiety Disorders, and abuse and/or neglect. Alternative explanations for conduct problems that should be ruled out include general medical disorders; any recent history of head injury, seizure, or exposure to known neurotoxins; and Psychotic Disorders. The next Application Note summarizes all of these considerations.

Behavior rating scales completed by parents and teachers can be helpful in establishing the occurrence of disruptive behaviors at frequencies beyond the normal range for given age groups by gender. Differential diagnosis among the various possibilities will require data from either clinical or structured interviews. In addition to the occurrence of major rule violations, another critical feature to be considered in regard to Conduct Disorder is that what is being sought is a *pattern* of behavior, not the occurrence of isolated acts, even if such acts are very serious. In practice, any real questions about a diagnosis of Conduct Disorder are almost always resolved by the passage of time. Youngsters with Conduct Disorder are pathologically unable to control their own behavior, even when they clearly recognize that it is in their own best interest to do so.

If the problems with oppositional behavior have not reached the intensity of major rule violations, then the primary differential diagnosis will be between Oppositional Defiant Disorder and Other Specified or Unspecified Disruptive, Impulse-Control, and Conduct Disorder. As discussed in the next DSM-IV-TR Note, a diagnosis of Conduct Disorder can now be made concurrently with a diagnosis of Oppositional Defiant Disorder; this change reflects a distinction between Oppositional Defiant Disorder as a disorder of emotion regulation deficits and Conduct Disorder as a disorder reflecting aggressive, deceitful behavior. This distinction also has implications for school psychologists. That is, it provides greater justification for eligibility of children with Oppositional Defiant Disorder under the special education category of emotional disturbance given its underlying conceptualization as a disorder of emotion dysregulation. Furthermore, it more squarely situates youth with only aggressive, destructive behavior outside the purview of special education services because of "social maladjustment." As noted by Biederman and colleagues (1996), the boundaries between these two classifications can be especially difficult to delineate, but this new rule allows for dual diagnosis of Oppositional Defiant Disorder and Conduct Disorder. Thus, it requires the examiner to review the criteria for both disorders and apply each when appropriate. A case that clearly meets criteria for Oppositional Defiant Disorder and includes only one symptom of Conduct Disorder may be best classified as Oppositional Defiant Disorder, with supplemental notation of the most serious symptom. A case of Oppositional Defiant Disorder with two clear symptoms of Conduct Disorder may be considered for a provisional diagnosis of Conduct Disorder coupled with an Oppositional Defiant Disorder diagnosis. Consideration of the empirically demonstrated predictive power of individual symptoms can be helpful. For instance, the work of Frick and colleagues (1994) suggests that fighting and other forms of mild aggression are often associated with Oppositional Defiant Disorder.

DSM-IV-TR Note. Changes in DSM-5 for Oppositional Defiant Disorder

The diagnostic criteria for Oppositional Defiant Disorder have been updated from DSM-IV-TR to organize the symptoms into three core areas of behavioral concern: angry/irritable mood, argumentative/defiant behavior, and vindictiveness. The specificity of these symptoms was also improved in some cases (e.g., spiteful or vindictive behavior has occurred at least twice within the last 6 months). The coding note also provides greater guidance in terms of how to diagnose at different developmental levels, with decreasing problematic behavior displays as the child gets older. Unlike the previous edition, the DSM-5 criteria also indicate that other factors, such as gender and culture, be taken into consideration.

It is important to note that a major change in the DSM is the conceptualization of Oppositional Defiant Disorder relative to Conduct Disorder. Specifically, in DSM-IV-TR, a diagnosis of Oppositional Defiant Disorder was ruled out if the child or adolescent met the criteria for Conduct Disorder (or Antisocial Personality Disorder). In contrast, DSM-5 allows Oppositional Defiant Disorder and Conduct Disorder to be diagnosed together. This change is rooted in a fundamental difference in conceptualizing these disorders. That is, emotional dysregulation is considered the core of Oppositional Defiant Disorder, whereas aggression, deceit, and/or destruction of property are considered core to Conduct Disorder. In cases in which both patterns of behavior are present, a dual diagnosis of Oppositional Defiant Disorder and Conduct Disorder is appropriate under the DSM-5 diagnostic criteria.

Application Note. Differential Diagnosis for Disruptive Behavior Problems

Consider:

Conduct Disorder
Oppositional Defiant Disorder
Adjustment Disorder With Disturbance of Conduct
Bipolar I Disorder, Most Recent Episode Manic
Intermittent Explosive Disorder
Child or Adolescent Antisocial Behavior (not a Mental Disorder; appears in Other Condition That May Be a Focus of Clinical Attention)

In addition, consider:

Attention-Deficit/Hyperactivity Disorder
Substance Use Disorders (adolescents)
Learning Disorders
Intellectual Disorder
Communication Disorders
Anxiety Disorders
Abuse or Neglect

Rule out:

Other Medical Condition that may be associated with aggressive or disinhibited behavior
Any recent history of head injury, seizure, or exposure to known neurotoxins
Psychotic Disorders

Despite their high comorbidity, Conduct Disorder, Oppositional Defiant Disorder, and Other Specified or Unspecified Disruptive, Impulse-Control, and Conduct Disorder on the one hand and Attention-Deficit/Hyperactivity Disorder on the other are conceptually and empirically distinct diagnoses. Given their frequent association, evidence of either type of disorder should prompt a specific review to rule in or rule out the presence of the other.

We suggest the following heuristic for a school psychologist confronted with a child or adolescent exhibiting disruptive behavior problems. First, does the case present with the essential feature of Conduct Disorder? If Conduct Disorder can be diagnosed, this will take precedence over Adjustment Disorder and Other Specified or Unspecified Disruptive, Impulse-Control, and Conduct Disorder. Next, consider the criteria for

Oppositional Defiant Disorder, bearing in mind that the essential feature of Oppositional Defiant Disorder behavior disturbances is emotion dysregulation. If the child is at least 6 years old and demonstrates a persistent pattern of aggressive outbursts, the diagnosis of Intermittent Explosive Disorder should also be considered (see later discussion). If there is no pattern of Conduct Disorder and/or Oppositional Defiant Disorder, then consider whether the behavior developed in response to psychosocial stress; if so, Adjustment Disorder With Disturbance of Conduct should be diagnosed. Finally, if characteristic features of a Disruptive Behavior Disorder are present but none of the specific diagnoses are justified, a diagnosis of Other Specified or Unspecified Disruptive, Impulse-Control, and Conduct Disorder should be entertained. DSM-5 allows the examiner to provide specific details regarding the relevant criteria for the individual (for Other Specified Disruptive, Impulse-Control, and Conduct Disorder) or to leave them out with the application of the Other Unspecified Disruptive, Impulse-Control, and Conduct Disorder diagnosis. The latter diagnosis is especially helpful in time-limited exposure situations such as the emergency room.

An evaluation of attention-deficit problems, impulsivity, and hyperactivity should accompany these considerations. Given the high comorbidity between Disruptive Behavior Disorders and Attention-Deficit/Hyperactivity Disorder, the school psychologist should always consider whether the criteria for Attention-Deficit/Hyperactivity Disorder are met when reviewing a case presenting behavior problems.

SPECIFIC BEHAVIOR PATTERNS

Conduct Disorder

The symptoms of Conduct Disorder occur at a low base rate among youth (this rate is consistent with the seriousness/psychopathology of these symptoms). It is therefore not surprising that empirical studies indicate that these symptoms have high positive predictive power but low negative predictive power. That is, the presence of Conduct Disorder symptoms is highly predictive of other symptoms and of the syndrome, but the absence of a symptom does not predict absence of the disorder (Frick et al., 1994).

The approach to subtyping of Conduct Disorder in DSM-5 continues to be based on age of onset of symptoms. If at least one symptom of Conduct Disorder has been manifested before age 10, the Childhood-Onset Type is identified; if all symptoms develop after age 10, the Adolescent-Onset Type is specified. (An Unspecified Onset option is offered for instances in which not enough information is available to determine whether at least one symptom was present before age 10, and the three

DSM-IV-TR Note. Changes in DSM-5 for Conduct Disorder

The diagnostic criteria for Conduct Disorder remained largely unchanged with the exception of the addition of specifiers about limited prosocial emotions. That is, examiners are encouraged to indicate whether two or more of the following are present: Lack of Remorse or Guilt, Callous—Lack of Empathy, Unconcerned about Performance, and Shallow or Deficient Affect. Decisions regarding the presence of these characteristics must be based on input from individuals who have known the youth for some time (e.g., teachers, parents, peers), not just self-report. The other two specifiers (i.e., Onset: Childhood, Adolescent, Unspecified; Severity: Mild, Moderate, Severe) remain the same. Thus, the specifiers are:

- Onset Type: Childhood, Adolescent, or Unspecified
- With Limited Prosocial Emotions → Evidence of at least two of the following:
  - Lack of Remorse or Guilt
  - Callous—Lack of Empathy
  - Unconcerned about Performance
  - Shallow or Deficient Affect
- Severity: Mild, Moderate, Severe

As with the previous edition, examiners should consider both the number of symptoms and the seriousness of symptoms in determining the severity. Mild cases have to have few symptoms above threshold and cause relatively mild harm to others, whereas severe cases may either have many symptoms above threshold or cause considerable harm to others. Moderate cases fall between these two extremes.

subtypes have received their own specific ICD-9-CM and ICD-10-CM codes.) The Childhood-Onset Type is believed to be more strongly associated with aggressive behavior and with risk of later adult Antisocial Personality Disorder. There is evidence for the validity of this approach to subtyping, as well as evidence for the validity of subtyping based on pattern of social affiliation (socialized/group/gang Conduct Disorder vs. unsocialized/undersocialized/isolated Conduct Disorder) or on the pattern of aggression (impulsive/reactive/hostile/affective aggression vs. controlled/proactive/instrumental/predatory aggression; see Christian, Frick, Hill, Tyler, & Frazier, 1997; Vitiello & Stoff, 1997). The superiority of one typology over another has yet to be convincingly demonstrated. Each version of the DSM that has considered Conduct Disorder, from DSM-II (American Psychiatric Association, 1968) onward, has employed a different (but related) subtyping approach. For a discussion of changes made to this diagnostic category from the last edition, see the previous DSM-IV-TR note on Conduct Disorder.

For clients over the age of 18 years, a diagnosis of Antisocial Personality Disorder preempts a diagnosis of Conduct Disorder. Because a history of Conduct Disorder is required for the diagnosis of Antisocial Personality Disorder, all clients who meet the criteria for the latter have met the criteria for Conduct Disorder in the past and will presumably continue to meet them. Rather than artificially generating multiple diagnoses, DSM-5 resolves this situation with the rule that Antisocial Personality Disorder precludes a concurrent diagnosis of Conduct Disorder.

Comorbid diagnoses strongly associated with Conduct Disorder include Attention-Deficit/Hyperactivity Disorder, Learning Disorders, and (in adolescence) Substance Use Disorders. Youth with Conduct Disorder tend to use alcohol and other substances earlier, more often, and more intensely and to sample a wider range of psychoactive substances. Highly dangerous forms of substance use, such as inhalant use, have been associated with Conduct Disorder (McGarvey, Canterbury, & Waite, 1996). Other comorbid diagnoses seen with some frequency include Mood Disorders, Anxiety Disorders, and Borderline Intellectual Functioning (not a Mental Disorder). Nonspecific attention problems, lower tested intelligence in the normal range, and impulsivity are also commonly seen characteristics. A specific risk associated with Conduct Disorder in adolescent females is the risk of pregnancy and single motherhood (Zoccolillo, Meyers, & Assiter, 1997), which can have multiple short- and long-range implications for both the new mother and her child. In a child or adolescent with Conduct Disorder, a careful review of other areas of adjustment requiring impulse control is warranted.

Assessment of comorbidity in cases of Conduct Disorder is clinically useful because this appears to be one variable associated with course and prognosis for adult outcome. In general, young people with two identifiable disorders have more difficulty than those with only one; those with three disorders face more challenges than those with two; and so on. Lynam (1996) has argued on the basis of his research that the child or adolescent with comorbid Attention-Deficit/Hyperactivity Disorder or Attention-Deficit/Hyperactivity Disorder-like problems *and* Conduct Disorder or conduct problems is at much greater risk for chronic offending into adulthood and eventual diagnosis of psychopathy than the youth with only one of these serious behavior problems. Our own experiences have been that the combination of Conduct Disorder and Substance Use Disorders in adolescents shows a potent negative synergy: Each markedly exacerbates the maladjustment associated with the other pattern of problems. Similar destructive interactions can be observed in the young person who is burdened with both conduct problems and a Specific Learning Disorder.

Careful assessment of comorbid problems, even if these do not reach diagnostic criteria, can yield a much fuller picture of the child's or adolescent's struggles in the world and can allow for better anticipation of future complications.

Oppositional Defiant Disorder

Oppositional Defiant Disorder as defined by DSM-5 identifies emotion dysregulation as central to the diagnosis. This change from the previous version of the DSM draws a better distinction between Oppositional Defiant Disorder and Conduct Disorder and now allows for the dual diagnosis in cases that evince significant disruptions in emotion regulation and aggressive behavior. However, the stringency of the criteria continue to exclude from diagnosis a number of children with problematic behaviors that adversely affect their school, community, and/or home adjustment. Many of these children, as well as some of the similar mild cases of Attention-Deficit/Hyperactivity Disorder excluded under the pervasive manifestation requirement, will probably end up diagnosed with either the Other Specified Disruptive, Impulse-Control, and Conduct Disorder or the Unspecified Disruptive, Impulse-Control, and Conduct Disorder categories.

The evidence at this time suggests that not all children with Oppositional Defiant Disorder go on to develop the more serious Conduct Disorder. In fact, some children with Oppositional Defiant Disorder go on to develop associated mood or anxiety disorders, whereas others continue showing Oppositional Defiant Disorder and some improve to the point that the behavior no longer justifies a clinical diagnosis. Nevertheless, children with a history of Oppositional Defiant Disorder, especially if treatment effects are limited, should be occasionally reconsidered for possible exacerbation of the intensity and quality of their acting-out behavior. A subset of children who have been appropriately classified as having Oppositional Defiant Disorder *will* eventually develop Conduct Disorder, and with the new diagnostic criteria some will be classified as having both at once. Reviews of the available empirical studies suggest that Oppositional Defiant Disorder and Conduct Disorder are distinct patterns but are related: Oppositional Defiant Disorder tends to show an earlier onset than Conduct Disorder; a history of Oppositional Defiant Disorder is almost universal in children who are diagnosed with Conduct Disorder (but, again, not all children with Oppositional Defiant Disorder progress to having Conduct Disorder); and familial correlates of Oppositional Defiant Disorder and Conduct Disorder are reported to be similar, with Conduct Disorder showing a greater density of these variables (Lahey, Loeber, Quay, Frick, & Grimm, 1992; Loeber, Lahey, & Thomas, 1991). Identifying the most optimal sets of symptoms both to establish Oppositional Defiant Disorder and Conduct Disorder and to discriminate between them remains a challenge. The Conduct Disorder symptom pertaining to frequent bullying, threatening, or intimidating of others, for instance, may actually be more closely associated with Oppositional Defiant Disorder than with Conduct Disorder (Burns, Walsh, Owen, & Snell, 1997). In "borderline" cases in which this is one of the deciding symptoms, extra caution in reviewing the entire clinical picture is warranted. Some evidence suggests that children diagnosed with Oppositional Defiant Disorder largely based on displays of aggressive symptoms and with childhood-onset Conduct Disorder are at greatest risk for an eventual diagnosis of Antisocial Personality Disorder, whereas children diagnosed with Oppositional Defiant Disorder largely based on criteria related to irritability and/or mood are more likely to be diagnosed with an Anxiety or Mood Disorder later in life.

Intermittent Explosive Disorder

The chapter on Disruptive, Impulse-Control, and Conduct Disorders includes the classification Intermittent Explosive Disorder to identify discrete episodes of loss of control of aggression that are not typical of an individual's usual adjustment. The behavior in question is generally quite intense, leading to physical assault or destruction of property, and it is judged to be out of proportion to any provocation that occurred. Of critical importance is that the behavior stands in contrast to the client's normal patterns of adjustment or maladjustment—the aggression is not typical of this young person. It also requires that the behavior is not premeditated or instrumental. That is, a diagnosis of Intermittent Explosive Disorder would not be appropriate for an individual who is emitting angry outbursts to obtain a tangible object or is proactive or predatory (as is the case with Conduct Disorder). Other Mental Disorders that could explain extreme aggression (a Manic Episode, a Psychotic Disorder, Borderline or Antisocial Personality Disorders) take precedence over Intermittent Explosive Disorder and would have to be ruled out before this diagnosis would be appropriate. Similarly, any substance use or medical condition that could account for unusual aggressiveness would need to be excluded. There may be suspicious physical conditions or events—a history of mild head injury, for example—that cannot be conclusively linked to the acute aggressive episodes. But if a causal association between such a neurological event and an illness could be meaningfully argued, the diagnosis of Intermittent Explosive Disorder would not be made. The diagnosis, in the example of a brain injury causing aggressive acting out, would be Personality Change Due to Another Medical Condition, Aggressive Type. As this example demonstrates, the exclusion of alternative explanations is critical to the diagnosis of Intermittent Explosive Disorder. Based on DSM-5 criteria, this diagnosis may now be assigned concurrently with Attention-Deficit/Hyperactivity Disorder, Conduct Disorder, Oppositional Defiant Disorder, or Autism Spectrum Disorder provided that the behavior is beyond that which is typically displayed with these disorders and warrants additional clinical attention. (See the next DSM-IV-TR Note.) Overall, DSM-5 provides better defined criteria for this disorder than did its predecessor, and care should be taken to examine the specific requisites in relation to other possible diagnoses.

We recommend that examiners use due caution in applying this classification to children or adolescents. It should not be used as a "catchall"

DSM-IV-TR Note. Changes in DSM-5 for Intermittent Explosive Disorder

The diagnostic criteria for Intermittent Explosive Disorder in DSM-IV-TR could be described as cursory, providing only two descriptive sentences and a list of rule-outs without the specification of requirements in terms of frequency, intensity, or duration. In contrast, the criteria provided in DSM-5 offer much greater detail and direction for examiners. They also shift the language from conceptualizing Intermittent Explosive Disorder as a failure to "resist" aggressive impulses to a failure to "control" these impulses, granting that the behavior is a disorder of emotion regulation and that it is, in fact, under the influence of the individual. It further delineates that Intermittent Explosive Disorder is demonstrated through either verbal aggression or physical aggression not resulting in damage at least twice weekly on average for 3 months or three behavioral outbursts that result in damage to persons or objects in a 12-month period. Intermittent Explosive Disorder may not be diagnosed before age 6 (or the developmental equivalent). To distinguish it from other disorders, it requires that the outbursts not be premeditated or executed to obtain reinforcement (e.g., attention, desired toy). DSM-5 provides more thorough discussion of rule-outs. Like its predecessor, DSM-5 rules out Intermittent Explosive Disorder if the behavior is better accounted for by another mental disorder, but it also is more specific about cases in which a dual diagnosis is permitted. Specifically, DSM-5 notes that an Intermittent Explosive Disorder diagnosis can be made along with Attention-Deficit/Hyperactivity Disorder, Conduct Disorder, Oppositional Defiant Disorder, or Autism Spectrum Disorder when symptoms are more severe than is typical with these disorders and they warrant clinical attention in their own right. DSM-5 also adds that an Intermittent Explosive Disorder diagnosis is not appropriate for aggressive behavior displayed by children and adolescents diagnosed with an Adjustment Disorder.

for cases of violence that are not immediately understood. We have found several instances in which a more careful review of a youth's actual substance use resolved the question of possible Intermittent Explosive Disorder clearly in the negative. There are, nevertheless, instances in which this diagnosis would be the most appropriate fit, and it should be considered in cases in which "unusual aggressive outbursts" are reported. Additionally, a thorough medical evaluation of the youth would be prudent, given the association of explosive behavior with a number of neurological disorders and the need to exclude these as explanations.

Adjustment Disorder With Disturbance of Conduct

An Adjustment Disorder With Disturbance of Conduct diagnosis requires two initial features: (1) identification of an apparent functional relationship between identified situational stress and the development of behavior problems (in this case, problems of conduct) and (2) a symptom picture of conduct problems that does not meet criteria for any specific syndrome or disorder. Failure to meet either of these conditions invalidates this diagnosis. An additional consideration is that this diagnosis is usually only maintained for a limited period of time. In DSM-III and DSM-III-R, a diagnosis of Adjustment Disorder was valid for only 6 months in children and adults; this was inconsistent with clinical experience and the empirical literature (Newcorn & Strain, 1992). As was the case with DSM-IV, DSM-5 is much less rigid than previous editions in the duration exclusion of Adjustment Disorder diagnoses, but the conceptualization clearly remains that of a transient disorder. Prolonged problems should prompt reconsideration of the most appropriate diagnosis. If the behavior problems persist more than 6 months after termination of the precipitating stressor, the diagnosis is no longer appropriate.

Other Specified or Unspecified Disruptive, Impulse-Control, and Conduct Disorder

DSM-5 increases the examiners' flexibility in dealing with classification problems by providing two additional, similar categories: Other Specified Disruptive, Impulse-Control, and Conduct Disorder and Unspecified Disruptive, Impulse-Control, and Conduct Disorder. Potential uses of these categories include cases in which young people present with evidence of acting out but the available data support only two symptoms of Conduct Disorder (at least three are required for diagnosis) or in which the pattern of difficulties cannot be documented over the required 12-month period (with at least one symptom in the last 6 months). The Unspecified category is useful when insufficient information is available for another diagnosis. Given the disturbing tendencies of conduct problems to persist and grow worse over time, examiners can expect that many cases assigned an initial diagnosis of Other Specified Disruptive, Impulse-Control, and Conduct Disorder will qualify for a more specific diagnosis (Conduct Disorder or Oppositional Defiant Disorder) as subsequent data are collected.

12

Problems with Impulse Control

OVERVIEW

As discussed in the previous chapter, behavior problems are one of the most commonly faced issues in schools. Beyond conduct problems, another major pattern of behavior problems is difficulties with cognitive focus, impulse control, and responding to situational constraints on behavior. Difficulties with focusing and shifting attention, impulse regulation, and self-control are often conceptualized in the literature as impairments in executive functioning and are a common source of frustration for teachers, parents, and the children themselves. (See the Author Commentary note.) A major and well-recognized syndrome is the experience of inattention, impulsivity–hyperactivity, or the combination of the two (DuPaul, Stoner, & O'Reilly, 2014). These symptoms are captured in the DSM-5 diagnosis of Attention-Deficit/Hyperactivity Disorder.

Author Commentary. Sympathy for Thursday's Child

Most readers of this book will have heard the children described in this chapter referred to as "the reason you will be sorry you ever chose to enter [fill in your own profession here: teaching, counseling, school psychology, etc.]." No question about it: Working with children with impulse-control and attention deficits can be incredibly challenging and often frustrating for the adults attempting to care for and educate them. It can be helpful to remind ourselves from time to time that these children are typically not being willfully disobedient, disruptive, or destructive. They are usually being quite honest when they tell us they "just forgot" to put the lid on the blender before turning it on or thought that drying out the wet cell phone in the microwave was a good idea. The literature and our own experiences suggest that many of these children suffer a great deal of peer and adult rejection and scorn because of actions with consequences they just did not foresee. Our impression is that many of these children awaken each morning hoping to themselves: "Please don't let me mess up again today." Our sense is that many of these hopes go unfulfilled.

ATTENTION-DEFICIT/HYPERACTIVITY DISORDER (ADHD)

Among the diagnostic and treatment questions most frequently presented to school psychologists are those concerning problems with overactivity, impulsivity, and distractibility, which are often diagnosed as Attention-Deficit/Hyperactivity Disorder. Multiple questions and controversies surround this topic, but the conceptualization of Attention-Deficit/Hyperactivity Disorder within DSM-5 appears to have significant relevance for educational settings (McBurnett, Lahey, & Pfiffner, 1993; see the next IDEA Note).

Within DSM-5, the diagnosis of Attention-Deficit/Hyperactivity Disorder focuses on clinical identification of one or both of two problem syndromes, namely inattention and/or hyperactivity and impulsivity, that adversely affect a child's adjustment in at least two major settings. The change from the single-setting formulation of DSM-III-R to the two-setting ("pervasive") formulation of DSM-IV was maintained in DSM-5 expressly to address a perceived overdiagnosis of "borderline" cases (excessive false-positive diagnostic errors), which is congruent with ICD-9-CM and ICD-10 definitions. The ultimate effect is to reduce the population of children formally identified as having Attention-Deficit/Hyperactivity Disorder, to increase the average severity of impairment of the population of children diagnosed with Attention-Deficit/Hyperactivity Disorder, and to increase the homogeneity of this population. The adjustments that were made to this diagnosis in the latest edition of DSM are detailed in the next DSM-IV-TR Note.

The diagnosis of Attention-Deficit/Hyperactivity Disorder has two presentations (as well as a Combined presentation): Predominantly Inattentive presentation and Predominantly Hyperactive/Impulsive presentation. The validity of the distinction between the two main presentations appears to be well supported both clinically and empirically, particularly for school-age children (Bauermeister, Canino, Polanczyk, & Rohde, 2010; Lahey, Schaughency, Hynd, Carlson, & Nieves, 1987). If the child meets the criteria for both Predominantly Inattentive presentation and

IDEA Note. Attention-Deficit/Hyperactivity Disorder and IDEA

Despite discussion of its possible inclusion, Attention-Deficit/Hyperactivity Disorder was not specifically identified as a separate category in the list of qualifying conditions in the definition of "children with disabilities" in the 1990 revision that transformed Part B of the Education of the Handicapped Act (Public Law 94-142) into IDEA (Public Law 101-476). It was the position of the U.S. Department of Education that Attention-Deficit/Hyperactivity Disorder did not need to be added as a separate disability, because children who need special services may be eligible for such services under the "other health impairment" category if their attention deficits handicap their educational performance (Davila, Williams, & MacDonald, 1991, pp. 2–3). Also, the symptoms of Attention-Deficit/Hyperactivity Disorder may meet the eligibility criteria for other mandated categories: "specific learning disability" or "seriously emotionally disturbed" (Davila et al., 1991, p. 3). Thus, if the symptoms of Attention-Deficit/Hyperactivity Disorder impair children's learning, the children may qualify for special education and/or other services under several existing categories. However, the diagnosis of Attention-Deficit/Hyperactivity Disorder, per se, does not qualify a child for inclusion under the provisions of IDEA (Davila et al., 1991, p. 4); only if the symptoms are severe enough for the child to meet the definition of "handicapped person" will he or she be eligible for services (Davila et al., 1991, p. 5). It is interesting to consider that the same argument could have been made about either "autism" or "traumatic brain injury," but these conditions were identified as separate categories in the list of qualifying conditions in IDEA. Students with Attention-Deficit/Hyperactivity Disorder who do not qualify for special education services under IDEA may qualify for accommodations under the Americans with Disabilities Act, Section 504, within the general education program.

DSM-IV-TR Note. Changes to DSM-5 for Attention-Deficit/Hyperactivity Disorder

The specific listing of symptoms within the diagnostic criteria for Attention-Deficit/Hyperactivity Disorder has not changed; however, several other changes to the determination did. For example, its location in the book changed: Attention-Deficit/Hyperactivity Disorder is identified as a neurodevelopmental disorder in DSM-5, not as a Disorder Usually First Diagnosed in Infancy, Childhood, or Adolescence, as it was in DSM-IV-TR. A few important changes were also made with regard to development. First, the age of onset was raised from 7 years to 12 years. In addition, a developmental adjustment was made to the criteria: Only five symptoms (rather than six) are required to diagnose an adolescent or adult. Finally, the specifiers were updated. Specifiers for subtype were changed to presentations (i.e., Combined, Predominantly Inattentive, Predominantly Hyperactive/Impulsive). The specifier "In Partial Remission" remains, and a severity specifier was added (i.e., Mild, Moderate, Severe). Minimal guidance is provided in determining severity.

Predominantly Hyperactive/Impulsive presentation, then the diagnosis of Combined presentation is made. In evaluating possible attention deficits without hyperactivity (Attention-Deficit/Hyperactivity Disorder, Predominantly Inattentive presentation), it is worth considering two symptoms that are not included in the DSM-5 criterion list: "often drowsy and sluggish" and "often daydreams." Both have high positive predictive power (actually better than many of the symptoms on the criterion list), but they have low negative predictive power; in other words, their absence is of little informative value (Frick et al., 1994; Skirbekk, Hansen, Oerbeck, & Kristensen, 2011). With regard to the Predominantly Hyperactive/Impulsive presentation, the symptoms of running around and climbing excessively and of acting as if driven by a motor have consistently shown high predictive value. Evidence of this characteristic strongly suggests Predominantly Hyperactive/Impulsive Attention-Deficit/Hyperactivity Disorder, but its absence does not connote the absence of Attention-Deficit/Hyperactivity Disorder (Frick et al., 1994). In contrast, the symptoms of inattention may be relatively nonspecific symptoms of a child behavior disorder (Halperin, Matier, Bedi, Sharma, & Newcorn, 1992) and are of little help in differentiating among Attention-Deficit/Hyperactivity Disorder, the Disruptive Behavior Disorders, Mood Disorders, Anxiety Disorders, and Psychotic Disorders. Children with an inattentive presentation may also be socially isolated, perhaps because of their difficulty attending to social cues (King et al., 2009).

The changes in formulation of Attention-Deficit/Hyperactivity Disorder in DSM-IV (that were maintained in DSM-IV-TR and DSM-5) appear to have met the goals of reducing the heterogeneity of the population diagnosed with this disorder, providing specific criteria for the Predominantly Inattentive presentation that are supported by empirical research, and identifying more impaired girls and preschool children (Lahey et al., 1994). The return to a differentiation between distractible–inattentive and hyperactive–impulsive syndromes is well supported (Bauermeister et al., 2010; Sabatino & Vance, 1994) and appears to have been well received within school systems (Erk, 1995; Gaub & Carlson, 1997). However, questions regarding associated risks and relationships of the Attention-Deficit/Hyperactivity Disorder presentations remain. Power and DuPaul (1996a) wonder whether the Predominantly Hyperactive/Impulsive presentation may not functionally operate to identify younger children who are at risk for eventually "exhibit[ing] the full symptomatic picture of the Combined type" (p. 291).

The changes in formulation of Attention-Deficit/Hyperactivity Disorder in DSM-5 from that presented in DSM-IV-TR are minimal. Indeed, the symptom list for Attention-Deficit/Hyperactivity Disorder is identical to that presented in DSM-IV-TR, although there are some other important changes to the diagnostic criteria (see preceding DSM-IV-TR Note), particularly the increase in age from 7 to 12 years for symptom presentation. According to Frances (2010), this change is likely to increase the number of youth diagnosed with Attention-Deficit/Hyperactivity Disorder.

Efforts certainly have been directed at making the category of Attention-Deficit/Hyperactivity Disorder useful and acceptable within a school setting (McBurnett et al., 1993). Despite these accomplishments, concerns about the high heterogeneity of diagnosed populations remain (Baumgaertel, Wolraich, & Dietrich, 1995). Disagreement also persists regarding the role of clinical judgment, possible bias, and the role of developmentally adjusted norms in the diagnosis of Attention-Deficit/Hyperactivity Disorder (Power & DuPaul, 1996b). Like its predecessor, DSM-5 does not address how the clinical information upon which to base a diagnosis of Attention-Deficit/Hyperactivity Disorder is to be gathered. Some authorities strongly recommend the use of behavior rating scales with age- and gender-appropriate norms (e.g., Barkley, 1990, 1991). We find such instruments invaluable in the assessment of Attention-Deficit/Hyperactivity Disorder and related disorders and have provided guidance for using them and other assessment methods within a multi-tiered system of supports (Tobin, Schneider, & Landau, 2014). DSM-5 does specify that the frequency and intensity of symptoms must be present "to a degree that is *inconsistent with developmental level* and that negatively impacts directly on social and academic/occupational activities" (p. 60; emphasis added). The text points out diagnostic difficulties associated with age-appropriate behaviors in active children, as well as with the need to consider the behaviors from the reference point of the child's mental age in children with Intellectual Disability. Although the examiner is free to make these comparisons in whatever manner seems appropriate, the use of age-graded norms certainly facilitates decision making. It is necessary to remember, however, that behavioral rating scales and decision rules can inform the examiner but do not reduce his or her ultimate responsibility. Behavior rating scales are not without their own problems, especially in terms of possible subcultural differences among populations of youth (Reid, 1995). The position of DSM-5, though a source of consternation to some, is clear on this point: It is the clinical judgment of the professional examiner that establishes the presence of symptoms to support a diagnosis of Attention-Deficit/Hyperactivity Disorder (or, indeed, of any mental disorder or other condition).

As noted previously, another continuing issue of contention regarding diagnosis of Attention-Deficit/Hyperactivity Disorder concerns the age-of-onset criterion. DSM-5 requires that at least "some" symptoms of Attention-Deficit/Hyperactivity Disorder must have been present and caused impairment before the child reached the age of 12 years. This criterion is a change from previous editions of the DSM. Previous editions required onset of Attention-Deficit Disorder (DSM-III) and Attention-Deficit/Hyperactivity Disorder (DSM-III-R, DSM-IV, and DSM-IV-TR), before age 7; there was no age-of-onset expectation specified for the Hyperkinetic Reaction of Childhood (or Adolescence) of DSM-II. Note that this requirement is not that the child have met full criteria for a diagnosis of Attention-Deficit/Hyperactivity Disorder prior to age 12—only that some characteristics were evident and had discernible negative repercussions in the child's life prior to this age. For most child clinical presentations of Attention-Deficit/Hyperactivity Disorder, this criterion is of minor significance. In the majority of cases, Attention-Deficit/Hyperactivity Disorder manifests itself early in children's development and is readily commented upon by various caretakers.

This change in age-of-onset criterion is likely to improve matters for those examining symptoms in adolescents and adults, particularly those with attention problems, some of whom were not diagnosed previously during childhood. This change may be especially helpful for children and adolescents with Attention-Deficit/Hyperactivity Disorder, Predominantly Inattentive presentation (Applegate et al., 1997). This increase in the age requirement will likely reduce but not eliminate the issues identified by Barkley and Biederman (1997), who argued that a set age-of-onset criterion is not well supported by scientific data and creates practical problems in the assessment of adolescents and adults being evaluated for Attention-Deficit/Hyperactivity Disorder. In particular, the accuracy of retrospective accounts by caretakers (some of which are given years from the time of interest) may be suspect, even when they involve rather dramatic behavioral symptoms. As Barkley and Biederman suggest, the age-of-onset criterion was significantly broadened, though it was not eliminated. For the present, however, the criterion is in place and should be considered as a necessary element of classification. The Attention-Deficit/Hyperactivity Disorder Not Otherwise Specified classification will be correct for the unusual case of a child or adolescent who currently meets symptomatic criteria for Attention-Deficit/Hyperactivity Disorder but for whom an onset of at least some symptoms causing impairment prior to age 12 cannot be established.

Frequent comorbid problems with Attention-Deficit/Hyperactivity Disorder include Learning Disorders, the Disruptive Behavior Disorders (Conduct Disorder, Oppositional Defiant Disorder, Intermittent Explosive Disorder, and Other Specified or Unspecified Disruptive, Impulse-Control, and Conduct Disorder), Mood Disorders, and (in adolescents) Substance Use Disorders (Pliszka, 2015). The various links between Attention-Deficit/Hyperactivity Disorder and Substance Use Disorders and substance use constitute a topic of continuing investigation and concern. Lynskey and

Fergusson's (1995) analysis of a large cohort of New Zealand children suggested that the association between attention deficits and later substance use was mediated almost entirely by the association between attention problems and conduct problems. Even if this conclusion is supported by subsequent work, the association between Attention-Deficit/Hyperactivity Disorder and conduct problems is strong enough to warrant careful monitoring of substance use in youth identified with Attention-Deficit/Hyperactivity Disorder.

The best understanding of the relation between Attention-Deficit/Hyperactivity Disorder and Bipolar Disorder continues to be a challenge for practitioners and investigators. In some cases, Attention-Deficit/Hyperactivity Disorder precedes by years the development of manic symptoms and may be an early developmental manifestation of Bipolar I Disorder. In other cases, Attention-Deficit/Hyperactivity Disorder and Bipolar I Disorder seem to be distinct but comorbid conditions. Faraone, Biederman, Mennin, Wozniak, and Spencer (1997), who studied a large clinical sample, concluded that comorbid DSM-III-R Attention-Deficit/Hyperactivity Disorder and Bipolar Disorder in children was familially distinct from other patterns of Attention-Deficit/Hyperactivity Disorder and might reflect what had been called "childhood onset Bipolar Disorder" in the previous literature. At this time, a reasonable recommendation would be for the school psychologist to maintain a sensitivity to possible signs of mania in children being evaluated for Attention-Deficit/Hyperactivity Disorder.

Although the clinical picture of Attention-Deficit/Hyperactivity Disorder may change, a high percentage of cases continue to manifest clinically meaningful symptoms into adulthood, with great personal morbidity in respect to academic achievement, social adjustment, occupational success, and individual accomplishment. Periodic reevaluations with respect to the current symptom pattern of Attention-Deficit/Hyperactivity Disorder, possible comorbid problems, and functional influence on the child's or adolescent's development and adjustment would appear necessary.

As noted earlier, the age-of-onset requirement for the DSM-5 diagnosis of Attention-Deficit/Hyperactivity Disorder is a major consideration, given the current popularity of and/or concern with this diagnosis in adolescents and adults. An appearance of Attention-Deficit/Hyperactivity Disorder-like symptoms in an adult or late adolescent without a history of similar problems going back to early adolescence may be more consistent with other DSM-5 diagnoses (e.g., Major Depressive Disorder, Bipolar I Disorder, Adjustment Disorder, Anxiety Disorders, and Unspecified Neurocognitive Disorder) or with some General Medical Conditions (neurological and systemic diseases). If alternative explanations are ruled out, the residual diagnosis of Other Specified or Unspecified Attention-Deficit/Hyperactivity Disorder may be considered.

Children who meet criteria for Attention-Deficit/Hyperactivity Disorder, especially the Predominantly Hyperactive-Impulsive and Combined presentations, should be considered with respect to Oppositional Defiant Disorder. We have observed a high rate of concordance between these two problems, consistent with rates often reported in the literature (Atkins, McKay, Talbott, & Arvanitis, 1996; Barkley, 2015). Conduct Disorder shows strong comorbidity with Attention-Deficit/Hyperactivity Disorder (Abikoff & Klein, 1992), as do Substance Use Disorders as the child grows into adolescence (Barkley, 2015). Biederman (1991) has argued that the heterogeneity of Attention-Deficit/Hyperactivity Disorder could be meaningfully reduced by considering the presence or absence of aggression as an important subtyping factor. At least some of the negative prognostic associations reported for Attention-Deficit/Hyperactivity Disorder may be mediated more by aggression than by Attention-Deficit/Hyperactivity Disorder symptoms (Hinshaw, 1992), and aggression can be used as a meaningful basis for distinguishing among children with Attention-Deficit/Hyperactivity Disorder (Roberts, 1990).

Learning Disorders also show a high association with Attention-Deficit/Hyperactivity Disorder (Hinshaw, 1992), perhaps especially with the Predominantly Inattentive presentation (August & Garfinkel, 1989). Halperin and colleagues (1990) have suggested a cognitive versus behavioral subtyping of Attention-Deficit/Hyperactivity Disorder. A careful screening for learning problems is always wise in children and adolescents diagnosed with Attention-Deficit/Hyperactivity Disorder. Tested intelligence may be an important prognostic factor in children with Attention-Deficit/Hyperactivity Disorder (Aman, Pejeau, Osborne, Rojahn, & Handen, 1996). Data concerning a child's mental ability can be noted in the clinical description, regardless of whether a codable condition exists.

Additional comorbid conditions frequently seen in children with Attention-Deficit/Hyperactivity Disorder are Mood Disorders and Anxiety Disorders. A DSM-III-R Anxiety Disorder has been reported to occur in up to 30% of children diagnosed with Attention-Deficit/Hyperactivity Disorder, and DSM-III-R Major Depression has been noted to co-occur with Attention-Deficit/Hyperactivity Disorder at the same rate (Barkley, 1991). Biederman (1991) has also suggested subtyping Attention-Deficit/Hyperactivity Disorder on the basis of additional diagnoses of emotional problems. In general, as noted earlier, the prognosis for two identified problems is worse than the prognosis for one, and the prognosis for three problems is worse than the likely outcome for two.

One concern expressed by Power and DuPaul (1996b) in their review of the Attention-Deficit/Hyperactivity Disorder diagnostic categories is that, because the medical model conceptualizes the problem behavior as a manifestation of a disorder within a child, this may reduce an examiner's sensitivity to environmental factors that influence the conflicts between the child and his or her caretaking situations. It is absolutely the case that DSM explicitly conceptualizes Attention-Deficit/Hyperactivity Disorder and all other Mental Disorders as disorders of the individual. It is not inevitable that taking such a view will lead one to ignore or minimize the powerful role played by setting variables and contingencies of consequences, but examiners are well cautioned to be sure to take these influences into consideration.

OTHER SPECIFIED OR UNSPECIFIED ATTENTION-DEFICIT/HYPERACTIVITY DISORDER

Other Specified or Unspecified Attention-Deficit/Hyperactivity Disorder diagnoses provide for the diagnosis of behavior disorders that show the essential features of Attention-Deficit/Hyperactivity Disorder ("a persistent pattern of inattention and/or hyperactivity–impulsivity that interferes with functioning or development"; p. 59) but that do not meet full criteria for Attention-Deficit/Hyperactivity Disorder. For instance, consider a child who shows 5 symptoms from the Predominantly Inattentive presentation criterion list and 5 symptoms from the Predominantly Hyperactive–Impulsive presentation list. Even though this child has 10 symptoms of Attention-Deficit/Hyperactivity Disorder, he or she does not show the requisite 6 from one group or the other. The appropriate diagnosis in this case is either Other Specified Attention-Deficit/Hyperactivity Disorder (if the examiner opts to specify the presenting criteria) or Unspecified Attention-Deficit/Hyperactivity Disorder (if the examiner chooses not to identify the specific criteria observed in the child). In all likelihood, further assessment of this child will turn up another symptom from one list or the other, at which time the diagnosis can be changed to the more specific presentation of Attention-Deficit/Hyperactivity Disorder. The examiner should note that this case is different from that of a child who at one time fully met criteria for one of the three specific patterns of Attention-Deficit/Hyperactivity Disorder (Combined, Predominantly Inattentive, or Predominantly Hyperactive–Impulsive), has shown remission of some (but not all) of the symptoms over time, and continues to show clinical impairment and/or distress secondary to the remaining symptoms of Attention-Deficit/Hyperactivity Disorder. This second child should be diagnosed as having Attention-Deficit/Hyperactivity Disorder, [Name of presentation], In Partial Remission.

It may also be possible to use the Other Specified or Unspecified Attention-Deficit/Hyperactivity Disorder category for individuals with an onset of symptoms after the age of 12. However, our experience is that this application is a very unusual development, and we recommend great caution in this practice. As Attention-Deficit/Hyperactivity Disorder has achieved popularity and familiarity in general publications, some individuals have seized upon it as an explanation of their difficulties. Attention problems are not unique to Attention-Deficit/Hyperactivity Disorder and in fact are common in many mental disorders—as are problems with productivity, difficulties in interpersonal relationships, and impulsivity. Only when the problems occur within the context of specific behavioral syndromes, cause impairment across at least two settings, and arise early in life does the diagnosis of Attention-Deficit/Hyperactivity Disorder usually apply.

OTHER IMPULSE-CONTROL DISORDERS

Also included in the DSM-5 chapter on Disruptive, Impulse-Control, and Conduct Disorders are Antisocial Personality Disorder, Pyromania, Kleptomania, and the residual cases: Other Specified and Unspecified Disruptive, Impulse-Control, and Conduct Disorder. Antisocial Personality Disorder is the only DSM-5 diagnosis that cannot be given to an individual under the age of 18 and therefore is not used except with older adolescents. The Antisocial Personality Disorder diagnosis is also included in the "Personality Disorders" chapter of DSM-5 and is discussed further in Chapter 15 in this volume on personality issues in youth.

Pyromania and Kleptomania in DSM-IV-TR were included in a grouping of Impulse-Control Disorders Not Elsewhere Classified. Both these diagnoses continue to be discussed in terms of (1) a building sense of tension prior to the act and (2) a sense of release, pleasure, or relief after the act. In our experience, actions that jointly fulfill these criteria are unusual in youth, whereas stealing and (occasional) fire setting frequently occur within the context of Conduct Disorders and/or delinquency, as well as in some perfectly typical children. Neither of these diagnoses is to be used if the behavior is better explained by a Conduct Disorder or manic episode. We urge careful review of any case in which these diagnoses were being considered.

We have never seen a case of Kleptomania in youth, either personally or in a professional setting. Without doubting the existence of this phenomenon, we suggest that it is rare and that more common explanations, such as Conduct Disorder, for simple stealing for functional reasons need to be firmly ruled out. We have seen this behavior in many children and adolescents as part of the problem picture. Stealing is a frequent problem in youth with Conduct Disorders and is especially difficult to deal with because (1) it tends to occur at lower frequencies than many other acting-out behaviors and (2) it tends to occur outside the presence of a caretaker. Such low-frequency, high-amplitude problem behaviors that occur often in community settings outside detection and monitoring are difficult problems for which to arrange consistent contingencies.

Pyromania, in the meaning of DSM-5, is also unusual in youth. Fire setting more generally is also a low-frequency, high-amplitude behavior that can occur as part of a Conduct Disorder pattern, as a delinquent act (which would be coded with the DSM-5 diagnosis of Child or Adolescent Antisocial Behavior found in the "Other Conditions That May Be a Focus of Clinical Attention" chapter), or as an experimental and sometimes tragic act by a unremarkable child. Careful assessment of the frequency, duration, circumstances, reported motivation, and experience of fire setting is called for in any clinical case of this behavior. Recurrent fire setting in general and certainly any diagnosis of Pyromania in particular will have a drastic influence on any efforts to place the child within many custodial or alternative living facilities. Many, perhaps most, child care placements view this as a safety issue with which they are not prepared to deal and will summarily refuse admission. Furthermore, this is a label that tends to follow a child through subsequent years, even after fire setting is no longer an issue. Because of the potentially serious consequences of both false-positive and false-negative diagnosis, this is a set of symptoms that all examiners need to be extremely vigilant and careful in evaluating. Fire setting is a serious but low-frequency problem in youth with emotional and behavior problems, and further empirical studies would be helpful. Further consideration of this topic can be found in Putnam and Kirkpatrick (2005) and Çelik, Aktepe, and Kocaman (2014).

OTHER SPECIFIED OR UNSPECIFIED DISRUPTIVE, IMPULSE-CONTROL, OR CONDUCT DISORDER

As with most of the other diagnoses in DSM-5, provision is made for externalizing behavior problems that do not meet the criteria for any of the specific categories recognized, and as with other problem areas the pattern is to provide two diagnoses. One of these, "Other Specified" identifies the reasons the pattern documented fails to meet criteria for a specific diagnosis in the group. The other diagnosis, "Unspecified," does not indicate the reason the case fails to fall within one of the identified patterns. As with other areas, both of these diagnoses are included within DSM-5 and within ICD-9-CM and ICD-10, and both have unique identifiers. Both require that the behaviors cause either significant personal suffering or distress *or* cause significant impairment in functional adjustment: That is, both require that the general requirements for a Mental Disorder be met. Both require that the basic problem be of a disruptive, impulse-control, or conduct-disorder nature (i.e., both require that the disorder be fundamentally the type of problem focused on in this group). The "Other Specified" category might be used to cover unique presentation or presentations falling short in duration or number of criteria. The text notes that "Unspecified" could include situations in which there is insufficient information available, although, if the exact deficits of the present record were spelled out, it would seem to move the diagnosis into the "Other Specified" category.

13

Highly Focused Symptom Patterns

OVERVIEW

A number of behavior problems commonly seen in children and adolescents revolve around single symptoms or circumscribed problem areas. Historically, difficulties with eating, sleep, elimination, movement, speech, and other focused disturbances of functioning were discussed as "habit problems." In DSM-II these were grouped in a section titled "Special Symptoms." From DSM-III onward, this heterogeneous grouping was divided among several categories: Several were addressed in the "Disorders Usually First Diagnosed in Infancy, Childhood, or Adolescence" chapter, whereas others were addressed in chapters covering specific problem areas (e.g., Sleep Disorders, Eating Disorders). In DSM-5, these disorders are further separated into freestanding chapters reflecting the affected functions: Feeding and Eating Disorders, Elimination Disorders, Sleep–Wake Disorders, Gender Dysphoria, and Paraphilic Disorders. Among the more commonly seen of these symptom patterns in school-age children are eating, elimination, and sleep problems. We discuss these disorders in this chapter, along with sexual and gender identity issues. They are presented in the order in which the first problem in each group appears in DSM-5.

EATING PROBLEMS

When disturbances of eating behavior, diet, and weight are being evaluated, one area of DSM-5 needs to be considered: the "Feeding and Eating

Disorders" chapter (pp. 329–354). This chapter includes Pica, Rumination Disorder, Avoidant/Restrictive Food Intake Disorder (new in DSM-5), Anorexia Nervosa, Bulimia Nervosa, Binge-Eating Disorder, Other Specified Feeding or Eating Disorder, and Unspecified Feeding or Eating Disorder. This arrangement is a significant improvement over its predecessor, which housed feeding and eating problems in three locations. Beyond this chapter, a brief description of Overweight and Obesity appears in the Nonadherence to Medical Treatment section of the "Other Conditions That May Be a Focus of Clinical Attention" chapter (pp. 715–727). Obesity and overeating are not considered disorders in DSM-5, but they may be addressed as Psychological Factors Affecting Other Medical Conditions, covered in the "Somatic Symptom and Related Disorders" chapter of DSM-5.

Specific eating behaviors (symptoms) may occur as primary or associated symptoms of several mental disorders. For example, significant weight loss or gain and/or decrease or increase in appetite can be a symptom of Major Depressive Disorder, Dysthymic Disorder, or Other Specified Depressive Disorder; appetite loss can occur in the context of Generalized Anxiety Disorder; and food rituals may develop in the course of Obsessive–Compulsive Disorder or Schizophrenia. However, when one primary focus of clinical attention becomes a recurrent pattern of difficulty involving food consumption and diet, an eating-related mental disorder should be considered.

Some Eating Disorders, such as Pica and Rumination Disorder, more commonly occur in early childhood, but they may be diagnosed across the lifespan. Beyond early childhood, they are more likely to present comorbidly with Intellectual Disability, Autism Spectrum Disorder, and/or other mental disorders. Other Eating Disorders, including Anorexia Nervosa and Bulimia Nervosa, tend to occur most frequently in adolescence, but with some significant incidence during childhood (and adult life). The most useful categorization of Eating Disorders in adolescents and adults, and the boundaries between these syndromes, continue to be actively investigated areas. For clients of all ages, the association of eating problems with physiological problems and medical instability should be kept in mind (Palla & Litt, 1988). Longitudinal studies continue to underscore the complexity of patterns of dysfunctional eating behavior, as well as the multiple associations with other patterns of emotional and behavioral maladjustment (Hall, Slim, Hawker, & Salmond, 1984). For a discussion of eating disorders as they relate to IDEA, see the IDEA Note on page 178.

SPECIFIC FEEDING AND EATING DISTURBANCE PATTERNS

Pica

Pica is the consistent consumption of nonnutritive substances for at least a 1-month period. "Scavenging behavior" is an alternative phrase occasionally used in the literature to describe eating nonfood substances. Historically, the nosological practice was to identify the substance eaten (e.g., "geophagia," eating clays or other earthy substances; "coprophagia," eating feces; "trichophagia," eating hair). Occasional mouthing, chewing, or eating of nonnutritive substances is not uncommon during the first 2 years of life and should not be diagnosed as Pica unless the behavior is problematic. Pica appears to be more common in developmentally delayed populations and may be more common in environments with limited stimulation. A major concern in cases of Pica is the risk of poisoning, especially exposure to lead, which is highly toxic. Pica can occur as an associated symptom of broad patterns of maladjustment (e.g., Autism Spectrum Disorder or Schizophrenia) or of neurological disorders (e.g., Kleine–Levin syndrome). In these cases, a separate diagnosis of Pica should be made only if the eating disturbance is serious enough to require formal clinical attention (e.g., a treatment plan, behavior modification program, or similar therapy focus).

Rumination Disorder

Rumination Disorder involves the persistent regurgitation and rechewing of food, typically in an infant or very young child. It occurs after a period of normal eating behavior and goes on for at least a month. There is often an association with general developmental delays. If there is an associated Autism Spectrum Disorder or Intellectual Disability, Rumination Disorder should be independently diagnosed only if it warrants focused treatment. Rumination during the course of Anorexia Nervosa or Bulimia Nervosa (see later discussion) is not separately diagnosed.

Avoidant/Restrictive Food Intake Disorder

Avoidant/Restrictive Food Intake Disorder is a new disorder in DSM-5. It is intended to capture infants and children who would have previously been diagnosed with Feeding Disorder of Infancy or Early Childhood under DSM-IV-TR, as well as individuals of all ages who do not eat or are extremely limited in their oral food intake. Individuals meeting the diagnostic criteria for this disorder evidence at least one of the following: marked weight loss (or failure to make expected gains in childhood), nutritional deficiency, need for nutritional supplements, and significant inference with social functioning. Careful medical evaluation is necessary to rule out biological causes. When primary organic causes have been excluded, the possible contributing factors include the individual's characteristics, which may make caretaking difficult, as well as inadequate skills and knowledge or maladjustment on the part of the caretaker(s). Presentation may include irritability, lethargy, withdrawal, and low soothability.

Diagnosis of Avoidant/Restrictive Food Intake Disorder may be especially helpful in work with children: Bryant-Waugh and Lask (1995) found that 25% of referrals to an eating disorders clinic were not well classified by DSM-IV. The atypical patterns they found included "food avoidance emotional disorder," "selective eating," and "pervasive refusal syndrome" (Bryant-Waugh & Lask, 1995). These descriptors fit well with the diagnostic criteria for Avoidant/Restrictive Food Intake Disorder.

Anorexia Nervosa

Anorexia Nervosa reflects a restriction of food intake that leads to a loss of normal weight (or failure to gain expected weight over time) associated with a morbid fear of being obese or with behavior that prevents weight gain and a perceptual disturbance in body image. Anorexia Nervosa is one of the few mental disorders with greater female than male prevalence; the majority of cases are females. Onset of clinical Anorexia Nervosa is often in adolescence, but concerns with body image and weight often develop prior to puberty (Sands, Tricker, Sherman, Armatas, & Maschette, 1997). The previous edition of the DSM pointed out that the term "anorexia" (loss of appetite) is usually a misnomer; most women with Anorexia Nervosa do not report loss of appetite, but rather a much more powerful fear of gaining excessive weight. The popular image of the client with Anorexia Nervosa as relying on self-induced vomiting (the "two-finger restroom run") is also not completely accurate. Some individuals with Anorexia Nervosa do make use of "purging behavior"—self-induced vomiting and/or abuse of emetics, laxatives, diuretics, or enemas. As common or more common in our clinical experiences is the more prosaic behavior of restricting eating excessively, sometimes in association with high-frequency, long-duration exercise. What clinically identifies the young person with Anorexia Nervosa is a body weight below normal combined with fear of becoming overweight and distorted body image.

Bulimia Nervosa

Bulimia Nervosa is a pattern of disturbance in which the individual (again, usually female), though excessively concerned with body weight and shape, experiences periods of loss of control over eating. Huge quantities of various foods, often high-calorie foods, are consumed. Despite these "binge" episodes, the young woman maintains a normal body weight. Maintaining a stable weight despite periodic ferocious overconsumption requires a compensatory mechanism to rid the body of the excessive calories consumed; this is the "purge" half of the binge–purge cycle of Bulimia Nervosa. Self-induced vomiting; abuse of emetics, diuretics, laxatives, and/or enemas; excessive exercise; and total fasting may be used singly or in various combinations to discard the excessive calories consumed during binges. Bulimia Nervosa behaviors, especially the compensatory mechanisms used, are medically dangerous. One factor contributing to the mortality of Bulimia Nervosa (as well as that of Anorexia Nervosa when purging is involved) is sudden coronary arrest associated with the electrolyte imbalances caused by purging. Among the medical morbidities, serious dental problems associated with recurrent vomiting are frequently seen.

Behavioral problems frequently found in association with Bulimia Nervosa include depression and self-injurious as well as suicidal behavior. Greater substance use has been found in adolescents with symptoms of Bulimia Nervosa, and the combination of Bulimia Nervosa and increased substance use predicts impulsive acting out in female adolescents—attempted suicide, stealing, and sexual activity (Wiederman & Pryor, 1996). Personality Disorders may be more commonly associated with Bulimia Nervosa than with Anorexia Nervosa, and a comorbid diagnosis of Borderline Personality Disorder should be ruled out. Like Anorexia Nervosa, Bulimia Nervosa is a potentially life-threatening disorder. The clinical situation is complicated by the normal appearance of the young person, which impedes identification of this deadly pattern of maladjustment. In childhood-onset Bulimia Nervosa, associated problems of depression and poor self-image are reported (Bryant-Waugh & Lask, 1995).

Binge-Eating Disorder

Binge-Eating Disorder appeared in the categories proposed for further study in Appendix B of DSM-IV, but it is now included in the Eating Disorders chapter of DSM-5. Binge-Eating Disorder is a pattern of abnormal consumption, loss of usual sense of choice or control over eating, and distress. What distinguishes it from Bulimia Nervosa is the absence of dangerous compensatory behaviors such as purging, excessive exercise, and use of emetics, diuretics, laxatives, and/or enemas.

Other Specified or Unspecified Feeding or Eating Disorder

The residual category of Other Specified Feeding or Eating Disorder is used for clinical cases that do not meet the full criteria for a specific Eating Disorder or show other atypical patterns of eating. The Unspecified Feeding or Eating Disorder category allows the clinician to identify cases in which significant disturbances in feeding and/or eating are present but do not meet the criteria for other Eating Disorders and in which the clinician does not have enough information or chooses not to specify the particular symptoms.

Psychological Factors Affecting Other Medical Conditions

A final category relevant to eating problems, Psychological Factors Affecting Other Medical Conditions, can be used to describe cases in which emotional and behavioral difficulties contribute to overeating. Obesity is included in ICD-9-CM and ICD-10 as a general medical condition, but simple overeating is not identified as a Mental Disorder in DSM-5. If there is convincing evidence that psychological factors play a significant role in a case of obesity, this diagnosis may be appropriate.

CLINICAL CONSIDERATIONS FOR EATING DISORDERS

Strong associations are reported between Anorexia Nervosa and current or future Major Depressive Episodes, and we recommend a careful assessment of possible mood disturbance or Mood Disorders in a young person with an Eating Disorder. Suicide is one factor contributing to the mortality associated with Anorexia Nervosa, and suicide risk should be carefully evaluated. Both because of the medical complications associated with starvation (as well as purging behavior, if it occurs) and because of the risk of suicide, Anorexia Nervosa is a life-threatening Mental Disorder, and an identified case requires aggressive treatment. Anorexia Nervosa also commonly co-occurs with Anxiety Disorders. In older adolescents and adults with Anorexia Nervosa, there may also be comorbid personality trait disturbances or Personality Disorders. Obsessive–Compulsive Disorder and Obsessive–Compulsive Personality Disorder may be overrepresented in patients with Anorexia Nervosa, especially those with the Restricting Type (Thornton & Russell, 1997).

Although Anorexia Nervosa is usually discussed in terms of a female clinical population, it is necessary to keep in mind that 5–10% of reported

IDEA NOTE. Eating Disorders and IDEA

Eating problems seem to be frequent in older children and adolescents in our society, and surveys often report disturbing prevalence rates of eating disturbances that could be classified as an Unspecified Eating Disorder (Steiner & Lock, 1998). Despite this prevalence, however, eating problems come directly to the attention of school psychologists relatively rarely. We have seldom seen the issue of an eating disorder addressed in an Individualized Education Program (IEP). Eating Disorders are not one of the categories covered under IDEA; however, their symptoms and associated challenges may qualify a student under the "serious emotional disturbance" IDEA category. The rationale and documentation would be similar to that used for mood disorders (see the IDEA Note on p. 86).

cases are male. Furthermore, the proportion of males may increase in childhood-onset cases (Bryant-Waugh & Lask, 1995).

DSM-IV Note. Changes in DSM-5 for Feeding and Eating Disorders

In terms of diagnostic criteria for the feeding and eating disorders, much remains the same, yet several important differences were noted. One major improvement is that all feeding and eating disorders are now presented in one chapter. The DSM-5 diagnostic criteria for one disorder are identical to what is presented in DSM-IV-TR (e.g., Pica), whereas the criteria for most other Feeding and Eating Disorders reflect minor changes. Most noteworthy are the elimination of Feeding Disorder of Infancy or Early Childhood and the addition of a new category, Avoidant/Restrictive Food Intake Disorder, intended to replace and extend the former category. Here are some of the highlights of the changes by disorder.

Pica

No changes were made.

Rumination Disorder

The DSM-5 diagnostic criteria include a specifier, "In Remission," that was not present in DSM-IV-TR.

Avoidant/Restrictive Food Intake Disorder (New in DSM-5)

This category was intended to capture individuals who would have previously been diagnosed with Feeding Disorder of Infancy or Early Childhood under DSM-IV-TR, as well as those who are older and experiencing food avoidance or severely restricted food consumption. This category is distinct from Anorexia Nervosa and Bulimia Nervosa because it must occur in the absence of disturbance in perceptions of body weight, image, or shape.

Anorexia Nervosa

In DSM-IV-TR, this disorder includes the refusal to maintain body weight at or above "normal" weight for age and height, defined as less than 85% of that expected. DSM-5 focuses on the restriction of intake relative to bodily needs, leading to low body weight. It defines low body weight as "weight that is less than minimally normal, or for children and adolescents, less than that minimally expected" (p. 338). The diagnostic criteria no longer require postmenarcheal females to experience skipping at least three consecutive menstrual cycles. Both DSM-IV-TR and DSM-5 include specifiers for type: Restricting Type and Binge-Eating/Purging Type. DSM-5 has two additional categories of specifiers:

Remission (In Partial Remission, In Full Remission) and Severity (Mild, Moderate, Severe, Extreme). The latter is based on calculated Body Mass Index (BMI).

Bulimia Nervosa

The diagnostic criteria are the same for this disorder, although the specifiers for it have changed. Specifically, the Type specifier (i.e., Purging Type, Nonpurging Type) was removed and two new specifiers were added: Remission (In Partial Remission, In Full Remission) and Severity (Mild, Moderate, Severe, Extreme). The latter specifier is based on average number of compensatory behaviors per week.

Binge-Eating Disorder

Moved from the "Criteria Sets and Axes Provided for Further Study" chapter of DSM-IV-TR, Binge-Eating Disorder appears as a new disorder in the "Feeding and Eating Disorders" chapter of DSM-5. The criteria for Binge-Eating Disorder are largely the same, although the frequency and duration have been reduced from twice per week for 6 months in DSM-IV-TR to once per week for 3 months in DSM-5. DSM-5 also includes specifiers for Binge-Eating Disorder: Remission (In Partial Remission, In Full Remission) and Severity (Mild, Moderate, Severe, and Extreme). Severity is based on number of binge-eating episodes per week.

Other Specified or Unspecified Feeding or Eating Disorder Categories

Much like the DSM-IV-TR category of Eating Disorder Not Otherwise Specified, the Other Specified Feeding or Eating Disorder category captures subthreshold disturbances in feeding or eating. DSM-5 provides five examples of specifers for this category: Atypical Anorexia Nervosa, Bulimia Nervosa of Low Frequency and/or Limited Duration, Binge-Eating Disorder of Low Frequency and/or Limited Duration, Purging Disorder, and Night Eating Syndrome. The Unspecified Feeding or Eating Disorder category is intended for cases in which clinically significant disturbance in feeding or eating is present but the clinician either does not have enough information or chooses not to be more specific about the individual's presentation.

ELIMINATION DISORDERS

DSM-5 provides for the diagnosis of two defined Elimination Disorders: Enuresis and Encopresis. Beyond these two Elimination Disorders are two other categories: Other Specified Elimination Disorder and Unspecified Elimination Disorder. The former category captures individuals with symptoms of an Elimination Disorder that do not meet the full diagnostic criteria for Enuresis and Encopresis, whereas the latter category is used in similar cases when the clinician chooses not to specify which criteria are not met or not enough information is available to make a specific diagnosis. The criterion sets for Enuresis and Encopresis are clear and take cognizance of the functional distinctions supported by the empirical literature with respect to frequency of incidents, age of onset, diurnal–nocturnal pattern, and history of continence.

It needs to be stressed that Enuresis is, by definition, not caused by disease or structural abnormality (cases of organic incontinence). In other words, it is imperative that a medical condition be ruled out before considering a diagnosis of Enuresis. Although research into the etiology of "primary course" (no history of established urinary continence) Nocturnal-Only Enuresis strongly suggests that it does have a biological basis, it is distinct from urinary incontinence associated with infections and systemic illnesses. Both Enuresis and incontinence will come to the attention of teachers and school psychologists. It is important to ensure that a proper medical evaluation has ruled out possible organic causes. Apparent "Enuresis" may be an early symptom of juvenile-onset diabetes, as well as of sickle-cell anemia or related disorders. Although cases of organic urinary incontinence in children are rare (some estimates suggest that as few as 5% of all cases of voiding of urine into bed or clothes involve illness or structural abnormalities), ensuring that these cases are accurately identified and treated is a responsibility of all professionals involved with children. Similarly, medical explanations for symptoms of Encopresis must be ruled out before a diagnosis of this Elimination Disorder can be made.

In our experiences, school personnel consider Elimination Disorders particularly problematic. They are disruptive, embarrassing, and test the clinician's obligation to provide confidential treatment when symptoms are present in a school. For example, one of us was shocked to learn that she was publicly applauded in the school newsletter for solving a specific child's elimination problems. Fortunately these issues, assuming no underlying medical condition, are relatively easy to resolve with treatment compliance of the child and the significant adults in his or her life.

GENDER DYSPHORIA

Gender Dysphoria reflects a basic conflict between individuals' sense of themselves as males, females, or persons of ambivalent gender on the one hand and their assigned sex on the other. They may come to clinical attention at any age. Coding is based on the age of the client; Gender Dysphoria in Children and Gender Dysphoria in Adolescents or Adults have different

ICD-9-CM codes. There is also an Other Specified Gender Dysphoria category to cover a heterogeneous group of residual problems involving distress related to incongruence between an individual's experience and assignment of gender. Encounters with these disorders will be rare in the experience of most school and child clinical psychologists. Multiple clinical and social issues are raised by both psychological and medical treatments of gender dysphoria (Nordyke, Baer, Etzel, & LeBlanc, 1977; Rekers & Lovaas, 1974; Wolfe, 1979; Zucker, 1990). Beyond initial identification, a referral to a specialized assessment facility is usually the most appropriate disposition (Cohen-Kettenis & van Goozen, 1997). In working with youth with Gender Dysphoria, it is useful to be aware of this disorder's association with symptoms of internalizing behavior problems and with Separation Anxiety Disorder (see Bradley & Zucker, 1997). The next IDEA Note sets forth how Gender Dysphoria relates to eligibility for services under IDEA.

IDEA Note. Gender Dysphoria and IDEA

Gender Dysphoria is a highly specific and infrequent pattern of maladjustment in youth and is not found on the list of qualifying conditions for special education or other special services in IDEA. However, diagnosis may qualify for inclusion under IDEA for services through the "emotional disturbance" category. To be clear, it is not the experience of Gender Dysphoria, per se, that may qualify the child but the related disturbances in thoughts, feelings, and social relationships that might lead to the need for services under the emotional disturbance or other health-impairment categories. Both the short- and long-term consequences of Gender Dysphoria are severe and negative, especially for males. Young females may find their peers and adult caretakers more tolerant of their violation of sex-role behavior, but young males tend to meet with harsh rejection and social abuse. Careful attention should also be paid to assessment of suicidal thoughts and/or self-harm, as these tend to be frequent associated problems with these youth (Skagerberg, Parkinson, & Carmichael, 2013; Spack et al., 2012). The negative influence of ostracism and isolation on their social development can be profound and long lasting, extending to affect their social adjustment as adults.

PARAPHILIC DISORDERS

Paraphilias become matters of concern in adolescence. Paraphilic disorders reflect deviant sexual arousal, urges, or behavior. Several classical patterns (Voyeuristic Disorder, Exhibitionistic Disorder, Frotteuristic Disorder, Sexual Masochism Disorder, Sexual Sadism Disorder, Pedophilic Disorder,

Fetishistic Disorder, and Transvestic Disorder) are specified in DSM-5, and two residual categories (Other Specified Paraphilic Disorder and Unspecified Paraphilic Disorder) is provided for less common patterns (telephone scatologia, necrophilia, zoophilia, coprophilia, klismaphilia, and urophilia, to mention only a few). It is worth reiterating that the diagnosis of a Mental Disorder refers typically to a pattern of behavior (not an isolated act) that has significant functional consequences (clinically relevant distress or impairment). Occasionally a psychologist is consulted by a teenager concerned that "a friend" has had a dream that included disturbing sexual behavior. Whatever their therapeutic uses, dream content is not the basis upon which Paraphilic Disorders are diagnosed—much to the relief, usually, of the teenager involved. Wulfert, Greenway, and Dougher (1996) have drawn interesting parallels between Pedophilia and alcoholism, based on a functional analysis of "reinforcement-based disorders."

SLEEP–WAKE DISORDERS

Sleep problems are probably common in children, but they are not often the basis of psychological evaluations. The Sleep–Wake Disorders include problems with the quality, amount, or timing of sleep and abnormal behavior in association with sleep, sleep stages, or transitions. DSM-5 distinguishes ten major disorder groups: Insomnia Disorder, Hypersomnolence Disorder, Narcolepsy, Breathing-Related Sleep Disorders (i.e., Obstructive Sleep Apnea Hypopnea, Central Sleep Apnea, and Sleep-Related Hypoventilation), Circadian Rhythm Sleep–Wake Disorders (Delayed Sleep Phase Type, Advanced Sleep Phase Type, Irregular Sleep–Wake Type, Non-24-Hour Sleep–Wake Type, and Shift Work Type), and Parasomnias (i.e., Non-Rapid Eye Movement Sleep Arousal Disorders, Nightmare Disorder, Rapid Eye Movement Sleep Behavior Disorder, Restless Legs Syndrome, Substance/Medication-Induced Sleep Disorder). Another diagnostic category system for sleep disorders is the *International Classification of Sleep Disorders, Third Edition* (ICSD-3; American Academy of Sleep Medicine, 2014). Thorpy (2012) reviews sleep disorder classifications including ICD-10, ICSD-2, and (the then proposed) DSM-5.

DSM-5 includes discussion of the advances made in sleep disorder medicine, and it has organized the disorders in this chapter accordingly. As with its predecessor, the text of DSM-5 relates each of its categories to those in the *International Classification of Sleep Disorders, Revised* (ICSD-2; American Sleep Disorders Association, 1997). This classification system was published by the American Academy of Sleep Medicine and is an important reference for investigators and clinicians specializing in Sleep Disorders. The ICSD has recently been revised and republished as a third edition (American Academy of Sleep Medicine, 2014), so some of the correspondences have altered, but the effort to relate DSM-5 to other influential documents in specialized areas has been an important step forward.

Sleep problems that occur in association with other mental disorders are seen with some regularity in clinical practice, especially in the context of Mood or Anxiety Disorders. The independent diagnosis of an Other Specified Sleep–Wake Disorder is only made when the sleep problem is severe enough to warrant being a focus of treatment. The same stipulation applies to Substance/Medication-Induced Sleep Disorder.

A related phenomenon is "bruxism" (teeth grinding). Nocturnal bruxism is often considered under the general heading of sleep problems. In an informative review article, Glaros and Melamed (1992) offer the following definition: "Bruxism is the nonfunctional contact of the teeth, including clenching, gnashing, grinding, and tapping" (p. 192). Bruxism is usually of concern because of potential dental damage rather than worry over a child's or adolescent's psychological adjustment. Despite interest in stress as a contributing factor, the literature in general does not suggest mental disorders in most children who grind their teeth (Glaros & Melamed, 1992). Bruxism is identified as a mental disorder in ICD-9-CM (306.8, "Other specified psychophysiological malfunction, Bruxism, Teeth grinding"), but it is not included in DSM-5. Nocturnal teeth grinding could be coded as Other Specified Sleep Disorder if circumstances met the general criteria for a Mental Disorder. Diurnal bruxism can be recorded in your case formulation without a mental health diagnosis if the sole concern is dental. The case of bruxism illustrates the general point that, whereas all DSM-5 diagnostic categories have legitimate ICD-9-CM/ICD-10 diagnostic codes, the converse is not true. Several mental health and medical conditions are risk factors for bruxism—cerebral palsy, Intellectual Disability in general, trisomy 21 (Down syndrome) in particular—and treatment is often provided using stimulant medications (Glaros & Melamed, 1992).

14

Substance-Related Problems and Other Addictive Behaviors

OVERVIEW

The "Substance-Related and Addictive Disorders" chapter in DSM-5 has been fundamentally changed. The "abuse" and "dependence" distinction used in DSM-III through DSM-IV-TR has been abandoned and replaced with a single category of Substance Use Disorder. Substance-Related Disorders are divided into two broad groupings: Substance Use Disorders and Substance-Induced Disorders. The Substance-Induced Disorders present in the form of one of the other mental disorders but are judged by the clinician to be the direct result of a chemical substance, either a prescribed medication, an electively taken substance, or a toxin to which the client has been exposed. The substance use problems are then subclassified, as in previous editions, by the substance abused. An additional diagnostic category provides diagnosis of Gambling Disorder, currently the only behavioral addiction formally addressed in DSM-5. (A research criteria set for Internet Gaming Disorder, which has not been deemed a Mental Disorder, is included in the Conditions for Further Study chapter along with Caffeine Use Disorder.) Substance Use Disorders can be specified further by course/remission status and by severity (based on number of diagnostic criteria identified). There are additional categories for situations that reflect the direct consequences of substance use, such as intoxication and withdrawal.

As in other DSM-5 chapters, considerable effort has been made to provide expanded specifiers to capture more details of the clinical presentation.

As with previous editions, DSM-5 provides substance-specific diagnoses for Substance Use Disorders, as well as Substance-Induced Disorders, Substance Intoxication, and Substance Withdrawal. For the general child clinician, the Substance Use Disorders will be the most commonly employed substance diagnoses. Clinicians working in emergency services and substance abuse programs will more commonly see intoxication and withdrawal presentations, but all mental health professionals should remain attentive to these possibilities, as well as the possibility of substance-induced manifestations that mimic common mental health patterns. The text also alerts the reader to changes that will occur when the United States moves from ICD-9-CM to ICD-10. ICD-10 will combine substance-use and substance-induced aspects. For example, in ICD-9-CM, Withdrawal and Abuse are given separate diagnoses; in ICD-10 a single diagnosis would be given (i.e., withdrawal would always imply abuse).

The basic approach to Substance Use Disorders taken in DSM-5 focuses on a "pathological pattern of behaviors related to use of the substance" (p. 483). Criterion symptoms for reaching this determination are organized into four general areas: impaired control, social impairment, risky use, and pharmacological criteria. The number of symptoms and the threshold criteria for the 10 different substance use classes vary. Severity is based on the number of symptoms evident. The specifiers for "early" and "sustained" remission remain but are more specific for "early" (requiring at least 3 months of absent symptoms). "Sustained remission" remains the same as it was previously: at least 12 months absent symptoms. In individual cases the examiner would do well to consult the manual for the specific disorder, as a number of substance-specific adjustments are made to the specifiers. For example, with Alcohol Use Disorder, "In Remission" requires at least 3 but less than 12 months without symptoms ("early") or more than 12 months without symptoms ("sustained"), but an exception is given for "craving, or a strong desire or urge to use alcohol," and the "In Remission" qualifiers can be given even if craving persists.

DSM-5 retains the 10 classes of substances addressed in previous editions of the manual (see Table 14.1). The text does note that these "classes" of substances are not distinct. The authors argue that all substances used in excess share activation of the brain's reward system. This statement is probably true and tautological. Other criticisms could be made of this grouping, which seems to be based more on historical and cultural practices than on any coherent theoretical or pharmacological scheme. It nevertheless adheres largely to the conventions often seen in substance use treatment centers. It is worth the reader's being aware that caffeine use, although capable of producing intoxication and withdrawal, cannot be

TABLE 14.1. Classes of Drugs Associated with Substance-Related and Addictive Disorders in DSM-5

Alcohol	Opioids
Caffeine	Sedatives, Hypnotics, and Anxiolytics
Cannabis	Stimulants
Hallucinogens[a]	Tobacco
Inhalants	Other (or unknown) substances

[a]Hallucinogens are further divided into phencyclidine/similar-acting arycyclohexylamines and other hallucinogens.

diagnosed as a Substance Use Disorder; Caffeine Use Disorder is not considered a Mental Disorder, but it does appear in the Conditions for Further Study chapter.

In fairness to the authors of DSM-5, the classification of psychoactive substances is an extremely challenging task (Hart & Ksir, 2012). Substances can be classified by chemical structure (e.g., tricyclics), by one of more of their common physiological effects (e.g., selective serotonin reuptake inhibitors), or by one or more of their common behavioral or cognitive effects (e.g., antidepressants). The same substance can have multiple placements in many classification schemes, and different chemicals can be found under the same heading. The field of substance abuse treatment has attempted for decades to address basic definitional issues, and no proposed scheme has enjoyed universal endorsement or acceptance. DSM-5 represents the latest attempt by the American Psychiatric Association to bring some useful and practical coherence to discussions about problematic substance use. There is little point in debating the positives and negatives at this point. It has the advantage of continuing the framework of previous editions, which should facilitate some epidemiological work. It should be noted that when the examiner is aware of the specific substance of abuse (e.g., alprazolam), this specific information is given in the diagnosis, along with the code for the substance group:

305.40 Alprazolam Abuse, Mild [two to three symptoms]

rather than:

305.40 Sedative, Hypnotic, or Anxiolytic Abuse, Mild [two to three symptoms]

Similarly, when a specific substance of abuse is known but does not fall within one of the 10 specified areas, the diagnosis would name the substance while using the ICD coding for Other Substance Use Disorder (e.g., *305.90 Anabolic Steroids Abuse, Mild*).

OTHER ADDICTIVE BEHAVIORS

In addition to the Substance Use Disorders, the chapter on Substance-Related and Addictive Disorders includes one "behavioral addiction," Gambling Disorder. Gambling Disorder was included for the first time in DSM-IV-TR, and this diagnosis is retained. Other "repetitive behaviors" were not included in DSM-5. The text notes that other possible behavioral addictions (e.g., "sex addiction," "exercise addiction," "shopping addiction") lacked sufficient "peer-reviewed" evidence at this time regarding important parameters to be included. There is no mention of Internet addiction as another possible behavioral excess (although Internet Gaming Disorder is included in the Conditions for Further Study chapter), nor any discussion of how excessive masturbation (which probably also depends on activation of the brain's reward circuits) is different from gambling. There also is no discussion of how gambling differs from Kleptomania. Whether it makes sense to include behavior patterns in a chapter on substance disorders is, again, beyond the scope of this text. In basic outline, DSM-5 continues the broad categories of substance and behavior seen in DSM-IV and DSM-IV-TR.

COMORBIDITY

A confounding issue with many cases of substance use problems is comorbidity with other emotional, behavioral, and environmental problems. While frequent comorbidity is a recurrent issue in almost all areas of psychopathology, with substance use there are particular difficulties with untangling the roles of other psychological factors, situational adversity, and developmental and sociological trends. Substance use difficulties in youth tend both to be increased by other mental health issues and to exacerbate other mental health problems. A thorough assessment using multiple informants may help clarify the diagnostic picture, but it is often a challenge even then to obtain a clear understanding of the interrelations among emotional distress, situational opportunities and pressures, and the initiation, continuation, and exacerbation of substance use. Careful attention should be given to co-occurring depression, anxiety, conduct issues (both clinical and subclinical), and situational stressors. When comorbid substance use and other mental health problems are present, concurrent treatment of both areas of difficulty is often necessary for best results.

CONTINUING ISSUES IN THE DIAGNOSIS OF SUBSTANCE USE PROBLEMS IN YOUTH

Tobacco, alcohol, and illicit substance use is common in adolescence in the United States. Swendsen and colleagues (2012) reviewed national surveys noting that by age 17 about 78% of U.S. adolescents had consumed alcohol and that 47% drank regularly (defined by 12 drinks in a given year); that between 59 and 71% had tried cannabis; and that 4–6% had tried cocaine. Although adolescent drug experimentation is a risk factor, it is not a reliable predictor of clinically significant substance use problems continuing into adulthood; no single variable or theory can reliably predict who is likely to develop a Substance Use Disorder (Meyers & Dick, 2010). Some researchers have described youth who meet diagnostic criteria for alcohol dependence prior to 25 years of age as "manifesting a form of 'adolescent alcohol dependence,' which may represent a less severe form of alcohol use disorder than that observed in adults" (Caetano & Babor, 2006, p. 111).

Although we might all wish that young people would postpone experimentation with psychoactive chemicals until after their first quarter-century, when their brains are well on their way toward adult maturity, it is not a realistic position. We are a substance-using society. Every day many of us make free use of any number of biologically active substances to enhance the quality of our lives (e.g., legal stimulants, antihistamines, decongestants, blood pressure medications, sleep aids). Some of these (e.g., caffeine) are in such common use among adults and children that we do not even think of them as "drugs." Others are seen as "good drugs" (i.e., "medications"). We accept the use of "recreational drugs" (e.g., alcohol, tobacco, in some states marijuana) among adults and treat these as "status offenses" in youth. The fact that many forms of substance use are acceptable in our society complicates efforts to define substance abuse in all populations. This distinction becomes even more challenging to differentiate when we are confronted with the rapidly evolving patterns of use (and abuse) in teenagers.

DSM-5 provides some assistance in this challenging enterprise by placing an emphasis on the consideration of four broad areas of substance use influences: impaired control, social impairment, risky use, and pharmacological criteria. Focusing on the negative influence of substance use in the youth's life provides guidance to the clinician both in terms of diagnosis and as a basis for therapeutic discussion. But no solution is perfect: It is easy to imagine being confronted by a teenager whose illicit substance use comes to light incidentally, who claims no problems are being caused by this use, who meets no psychological criteria, and who maintains that his or her use of *X* is "no big deal." How many of us would be willing to ignore this situation? On some level professionals need to live with the ambiguity that we cannot perfectly identify which adolescents have clinically significant substance use patterns (we certainly do better with more intense levels of use), nor which adolescents are highly likely to continue to have substance use problems into adult life (again, we can do better with more severe, long-enduring patterns, especially with comorbid behavior and emotional problems, but even in these cases individual predictions are fraught with error). To certain substances, we may feel more confident assigning diagnostic weight (e.g., cocaine and nicotine are highly addictive; phencyclidine [PCP] and 3,4-methylenedioxy-methamphetamine [MDMA; Ecstasy, Molly] have potential for central nervous system damage), but there are risks to all substance uses (even the good ones we consider medication). Certain patterns of use may concern us regarding the youth's development or even safety (i.e., increased time and resources devoted to use and decreased attention to previous prosocial activities or friends), but adolescence often sees dramatic shifts in activities, interests, and associations. The age of onset is often identified as one of the most potent predictors of difficulty, and many of us have a lower threshold of concern for children than for teenagers. At the end of the day, there will be no alternative to a careful and thorough evaluation of the young person, his or her life situation, and how substance use is influencing his or her functioning for us to reach any meaningful substance use diagnoses in youth.

The major subclassification within DSM-5 remains pharmacological classification. This division creates some difficulties. Crowley (2006) points out that the cough suppressant Coricidin HBP Cough and Cold Tablets, referred to as "Triple C," has been abused by adolescents, but categorizing it is difficult: "Its main active ingredient, dextromethorphan, is a *d*-isomer opioid, active at the sigma opioid receptor but thought to have little affinity for the mu receptor. An active metabolite blocks NMDA [*N*-methyl-*D*-aspartate] receptors, as does phencyclidine. Clinicians and researchers have no current guidance on whether to categorize 'Triple C' with the opioid drugs or among the 'Phencyclidine or Phencyclidine-Like Substances" (p. 121). He also points out that popular "club drugs" may have mixed pharmacological properties.

One possibility to consider is that a single subtyping topology may not be the most useful direction at this time. Babor and Caetano (2006) consider the current state of affairs regarding subtypes of Substance Use Disorder and review characteristics of an optimal typology. The research they review suggests that for alcohol use problems a consistent pattern observed is two broad groupings based on vulnerability factors (e.g., family history of alcohol abuse, childhood behavior disorder) and severity (chronicity of use, age of onset, number of symptoms). Consideration of such two-factor models may be useful for clinical analysis, but it is not sufficiently supported, at this time, by empirical data to be codified into a diagnostic system.

And a final consideration for the weary clinician confronted with the issue of substance use and abuse in youth is this additional challenge: Even under optimal reporting conditions and complete honesty in our young client, he or she may be unaware, confused, or deliberately misled about what substances he or she has actually consumed. For anyone who has worked in an emergency room or medical setting, the frequent incongruity between reported consumption and the toxicology report is no surprise. Although some of this inconsistency represents deliberate minimization and denial, other instances seem clearly to represent "honest" but "non-veridical" reporting: The young persons have told us what they believe they consumed, but the reality is something different. In most instances in which youth engage in substance abuse, at some point they have had to interact with criminals or at least people who were willing to engage in criminal behavior. The reality that sometimes sellers of illicit substances misrepresent what they are actually selling is not a shocking idea. And even the supplier may be uninformed or ignorant of what chemicals are actually present in the product. Whereas alcohol, tobacco, and caffeine products (and in some states, to a degree, marijuana) are regulated, illicit substances are usually created in nonstandardized conditions. Even with actual medications, there may be quality control issues when they are obtained from illicit sources outside the country or through the "dark net."

Regardless of the classification system used, the most basic and fundamental principle of assessment for potential substance use problems in youth (as in all other populations) is to ask about it. Inquiring about tobacco use, alcohol use, illicit drug use, marijuana use (many teenagers and adults do not view marijuana as an illicit drug), medication use, and compliance should be a routine part of any psychological evaluation. Brief screening questions and probes can be used to minimize the amount of time consumed if substance use turns out not to be a significant factor (e.g., the CRAFFT screen for adolescents [Knight, Sherritt, Shrier, Harris, & Chang, 2002]; see also National Institute on Alcohol Abuse and Alcoholism [NIAAA], 2011). Undetected substance use problems are significant contributors to mental health and adjustment difficulties in young people. Clients can minimize, dissimulate, and lie, but many, even teenagers, if asked directly in a clear and nonjudgmental manner, will provide information on their chemical use if we just ask.

IDEA Note. Alcohol and Substance Use Disorders and IDEA

Alcohol and Substance Use Disorders are not disabilities covered under IDEA. These disorders could be covered under the Americans with Disabilities Act/ Section 504 if they significantly limit a major life activity, such as learning or attending school.

15

Personality Disorders

DIAGNOSING PERSONALITY DISORDERS IN YOUTH: CONTROVERSY AND CAUTIONS

The question of whether Personality Disorders actually occur in children and adolescents is a relatively new one and has generated controversy. The basic idea of a "personality disorder" is of a sustained pattern of rigid and excessive traits that compromises an individual's adjustment or functioning across multiple settings. The construct of "personality" is, of course, an old one in psychology, and its study has reflected the various concerns of groups within the social sciences. The idea that there are reliable, cross-situational consistencies in actions was challenged by some psychologists during the 1960s and 1970s (most notably Mischel, 1968), but in more recent formulations many theorists seem to accept some degree of consistency in human behavior, paralleling conventional ideas of personality. Cognitive-behavioral treatment approaches for Personality Disorders have further established this renewed acceptance of the concept of personality (Beck, Freeman, & Associates, 1990; Linehan, 1993; Turkat, 1990; Young, 1990), although a few behavioral theorists still do not accept the concept's usefulness (see, e.g., Koerner, Kohlenberg, & Parker, 1996). Personality disorders were originally separated from other clinical syndromes in DSM-III as pathological exaggerations of personality traits. This basic view is maintained in DSM-5, although personality disorders are no longer grouped separately from other clinical disorders with the abandonment of the multiaxial approach.

It is worth considering that personality diagnosis was possibly one of the most contentious areas in the construction of DSM-5. The manual notes that different viewpoints emerged, and essentially two perspectives are offered. In Section II (Diagnostic Criteria and Codes) of DSM-5, updates to the 10 personality disorder diagnoses from DSM-IV and DSM-IV-TR (plus Personality Change Due to Another Medical Condition and Other Specified Personality Disorder and Unspecified Personality Disorder) are provided. This coverage is essentially the same categorical model that emerged in DSM-III and was significantly influenced by the personality model of Theodore Millon. Section III (Emerging Measures and Models) of DSM-5 provides a section called "Alternative DSM-5 Model for Personality Disorders." This section presents a dimensional model significantly influenced by the five-factor model of personality that has been widely accepted in much psychological research. The text offers the positive take "it is hoped that both versions will serve clinical practice and research initiatives" (p. 645); but a more cynical view might be that a collection of the world's experts on this topic were unable to come to any consensus about how best to conceptualize, measure, or diagnose personality disorders. It might reasonably be inferred that some caution and restraint would be advised in offering too rigid or conclusive statements in this area.

DSM-5 defines "personality traits" as "enduring patterns of perceiving, relating to, and thinking about the environment and oneself that are exhibited in a wide range of social and personal contexts" (p. 647). A Personality Disorder is characterized by traits that are inflexible and maladaptive and that cause either significant personality distress or functional impairment (the fundamental criterion for a Mental Disorder). The dysfunctional pattern of a Personality Disorder must be evident across a range of environmental settings, consistent and enduring over time, and evident by adolescence or early adulthood. From this basic view of personality problems emerges the conflict inherent in using the Personality Disorder categories with children and adolescents. Explicit in the definition of a Personality Disorder is the belief that these excessively rigid traits should be manifested from relatively early in life (and should therefore be available for clinical diagnosis). Yet, from a different perspective, it can be questioned how much confidence we can ever have in a Personality Disorder diagnosis in childhood or adolescence. To what extent has there been any opportunity to evaluate how stable this behavior pattern will be across settings when a young person has usually experienced relatively few environments? And how can we speak of stability over time when the young person has lived but a small fraction of his or her potential lifespan? Probably the best empirical case for the stability and validity of a Personality Disorder category applied to children and youth could be made for Antisocial Personality Disorder—which, as it happens, is the *only* Personality

Disorder diagnosis explicitly precluded from use when the client is less than 18 years of age.

With the exception of Antisocial Personality Disorder, the Personality Disorder diagnoses are available for use with older children and adolescents. DSM-5 requires only that the diagnostic features must have been evident for at least 1 year in clients under 18 years of age (p. 647). Our recommendation, however, is for caution in using Personality Disorder diagnoses in youth (see also Lewis, 1996). Although indicating dysfunctional personality traits may be useful in understanding the problems of a young person and may set valuable targets for therapeutic change, the decision to conceptualize the problems of a young person as a Personality Disorder implies a stability that we think is often lacking in the development of individuals during their first quarter-century of life. We advise that, as part of making a decision about use of a Personality Disorder diagnosis, examiners consider not only the specific categorical criteria but also the general diagnostic criteria for a Personality Disorder (pp. 646–647). Perhaps the most useful heuristic is frequently patience: If a young person actually has a Personality Disorder, then the problems will continue, and even more evidence of the disorder's existence will accumulate. This reality does not mean that therapeutic efforts to enhance the young person's adjustment need be postponed. The evaluator can identify problematic behavior patterns and make these the focus of change efforts. If the behavior problems are resistant to these efforts, the case for a Personality Disorder is strengthened. If moderation is achieved and a better level of adjustment and functioning results, then the question is moot.

OTHER CAUTIONS ABOUT DIAGNOSING PERSONALITY DISORDERS

DSM-5 recommends caution in diagnosing Personality Disorders during active episodes of Mood or Anxiety Disorders because the symptoms of these disorders may "mimic" personality traits and may complicate the retrospective evaluation of a client's long-standing temperament. This caution seems well advised. The cognitive features associated with mood and anxiety problems may distort retrospective reports, and it is possible that the experience of interacting with a child or adolescent with depressive symptoms may influence the retrospective impression of a caretaker who is being interviewed about "premorbid personality features." Although the possibility of personality traits and potentially dysfunctional personality traits can always be noted in diagnostic impressions, we recommend that Personality Disorders not be based exclusively on data gathered during acute episodes of Mood, Anxiety, Somatic Symptom, or Dissociative Disorders.

Another consideration that must be given special attention in the potential diagnosis of a Personality Disorder is any potential involvement in substance misuse. The literature on the reliability of Personality Disorder diagnoses in adults strongly suggests the hazard of making such diagnoses during periods of active Substance Abuse or Dependence or during detoxification from Substance Dependence. In the absence of clear evidence of years of premorbid occurrence of rigid and dysfunctional personality traits prior to any active substance use by a child or adolescent, we recommend deferring any diagnosis of a Personality Disorder until after the establishment of a stable period of substance-free living. Nevertheless, significant associations have been reported between Substance Use Disorders and Borderline Personality Disorder in adolescents, and especially among Substance Use Disorders, Major Depressive Disorders, and Borderline Personality Disorder (Grilo, Walker, Becker, Edell, & McGlashan, 1997).

Personality Disorder diagnoses are often comorbid with other mental disorder diagnoses (Lewinsohn, Rohde, Seeley, & Klein, 1997). Personality Disorder diagnoses are also associated with greater distress and functional impairment in troubled adolescents (Bernstein et al., 1993). Finally, although some adolescent diagnoses of Personality Disorder are stable over time, many were not found to be evident at the end of a 2-year follow-up study (Bernstein et al., 1993). Considering the multiple indications that personality phenomena may be better conceptualized as traits than as types, there may be inherent limitations in a categorical model of personality pattern difficulty.

Given these preliminary considerations, let us now consider the three broad groupings of Personality Disorders within DSM-5: Cluster A (odd–eccentric), Cluster B (dramatic–emotional), and Cluster C (anxious–fearful). The next IDEA Note sets forth how Personality Disorders in general and the Cluster B disorders in particular relate to eligibility for services under IDEA.

CLUSTER A (ODD–ECCENTRIC) PERSONALITY DISORDERS

With the exception of Antisocial Personality Disorder, which by definition shows a childhood or young adolescent precursor state (i.e., Conduct Disorder), possibly the best evidence for the existence of Personality Disorder phenomena in youth can be marshaled for the categories from the odd–eccentric cluster of Personality Disorders: Paranoid, Schizoid, and Schizotypal Personality Disorders. All are described as possibly being first apparent in childhood, with similar manifestations and social consequences (peer rejection, teasing). A discussion of the role of this social isolation from possibly "corrective" peer feedback in the possible exacerbation of these problems is beyond the scope of this work, but it is clearly an area for further investigation. The available literature suggests that all three patterns in their extreme (i.e., diagnosable) form may be very stable. This conclusion is especially interesting in regard to Schizotypal Personality Disorder, which was originally conceptualized as a possible precursor to Schizophrenia but has since been discredited as such. DSM-5 points out the potential difficulty in distinguishing Schizoid and Schizotypical Personality Disorder from Autism Spectrum and Language Disorders and Paranoid Personality Disorder from Psychotic Disorders. The differentiation is based on severity of social impairments and restricted repertoire and pervasiveness of presentations over time and across situations. Although the general cautions about using Personality Disorder diagnoses with children and adolescents (discussed earlier) also apply to the Cluster A categories, this particular cluster seems to constitute areas of both valid clinical use and continued empirical investigation.

IDEA Note. Personality Disorders and IDEA

We are unaware of any cases in which eligibility for special education services under IDEA has been sought on the basis of a diagnosed Personality Disorder in a child or adolescent. Given the high reported comorbidity of other Mental Disorders in youth classified as manifesting Personality Disorders, it is likely that there are young people with Personality Disorders who are receiving special education or other services whose eligibility was demonstrated on the basis of the other presenting Mental Disorders. Nevertheless, given the disruptive nature of the Cluster B (dramatic–emotional) Personality Disorders, it is quite possible that one may eventually be identified as the primary or sole reason for a young person's need of special education services under IDEA. The nature of Personality Disorders—enduring, resistant to change, rigid, and nonadaptive—should address most of the basic requirements of the "emotional disturbance" category of eligibility.

The essential task of the school psychologist advancing such a case is to demonstrate the functional limitations manifested in the child's or adolescent's school performance because of these characteristics. This demonstration may or may not pose a challenge. For some young people with personality trait disturbances, the interference with their school achievement is evident to all observers. Yet it has been our experience that some adolescents showing borderline traits may actually do their best in academic activities. The structure and attention available in schoolwork may help them constrain their rigid and extreme temperament and achieve a degree of confidence and success not seen in other areas of their lives. The ongoing discussion of including social maladjustment problems in IDEA should bring even more attention to this question of how Personality Disorders should be treated under IDEA.

CLUSTER B (DRAMATIC–EMOTIONAL) PERSONALITY DISORDERS

Antisocial Personality Disorder

As noted earlier, Antisocial Personality Disorder cannot be diagnosed prior to age 18; by definition, however, there is preexisting Conduct Disorder before the age of 15. We have found it valuable to note in adolescent classifications those cases in which continuation of the observed pattern of antisocial behavior will justify a clinical diagnosis of Antisocial Personality Disorder when the individual reaches the age of 18.

Borderline Personality Disorder

The usefulness of conceptualizing difficult-to-deal-with youth as manifesting Borderline Personality Disorder will undoubtedly continue to be actively debated (Bleiberg, 1994; Lewis, 1996), especially because several empirically validated treatments for this disorder are available. The Substance Abuse and Mental Health Services Administration (SAMHSA; 2015) National Registry of Evidence-based Programs and Practices (NREPP) currently lists four empirically supported interventions for Borderline Personality Disorder: Dialectical Behavior Therapy, Systems Training for Emotional Predictability and Problem Solving (STEPPS), Dynamic Deconstruction Psychotherapy, and Psychoeducational Multifamily Groups. In our experiences, this Personality Disorder category is most commonly evoked in classifying adolescents—especially those with chronic problems, poor response to treatments, and demanding personality features. Yet, despite the concern over heterogeneity of populations, the possibility that "borderline" characteristics or even diagnoses of Borderline Personality Disorder in children are not good predictors of diagnosis of this disorder in adults (Lewis, 1996), and the worry that we may be doing little more than applying a prejudicial label to particularly troublesome clients, there is some evidence that Borderline Personality Disorder may be a viable diagnostic category for adolescents (Ludolph et al., 1990; Westen, Ludolph, Lerner, Ruffins, & Wiss, 1990). A study by Guzder, Paris, Zelkowitz, and Marchessault (1996) on risk factors for borderline pathology in children is worth considering; this group found that sexual abuse, physical abuse, severe neglect, and parental substance abuse or criminal behavior differentiated between their groups of children with and without a diagnosis of Borderline Personality Disorder (made with the Child Diagnostic Interview for Borderlines). The Grilo and colleagues (1997) study cited previously reported higher rates of Borderline Personality Disorder in hospitalized adolescents with diagnoses of Major Depressive Disorder, of a Substance Use Disorder, and especially with a combination of Major Depressive Disorder and a Substance Use Disorder.

We have sometimes found it useful to identify borderline traits being displayed by an adolescent. These traits can be identified, listed, or discussed in a case conceptualization; however, we have had few occasions to feel confident about applying a DSM-5 diagnosis of Borderline Personality Disorder to an adolescent. Goldman, D'Angelo, Demaso, and Mezzacappa (1992) suggest modifications of the DSM-III-R criterion set for Borderline Personality Disorder to make it more applicable to adolescents. We think the best course of action, if a teenager is identified by such a modified criterion set but does not meet the DSM-5 criteria, is to make a diagnosis of Other Specified Personality Disorder and explain that the young person does meet an experimental set of diagnostic criteria. We still advise great caution regarding the utility of a conceptualization of Borderline Personality Disorder in adolescents because this diagnosis in youth seems to be more strongly associated with other mental health diagnoses than with Personality Disorder diagnoses at follow-up (Lewis, 1996).

Another diagnostic concern is that multiple mental disorders may occur in association with Borderline Personality Disorder. Concurrent Mood Disorders, Anxiety Disorders, Substance Use Disorders, Attention-Deficit/Hyperactivity Disorder, Conduct Disorder, and (in a few cases) Dissociative Disorders may occur. The combination of Borderline Personality Disorder with Depressive Disorders may be especially dangerous with respect to suicide risk (Pfeffer, 1992). Repeated instances of nonlethal, self-injurious behaviors are almost pathognomonic for Borderline Personality Disorder (Linehan, 1993), but some care must be exercised to differentiate between these symptoms and various subculturally supported "deviant behaviors of youth," such as nonprofessional tattooing, body piercing, decorative scarring, and the like, which can also be seen both in youth with Conduct Disorders and in extremely rebellious or idiosyncratic (but not mentally ill) youth.

A final concern about the Borderline Personality Disorder diagnostic category is the name of this entity. The term "borderline personality" is a holdover from the original psychoanalytic conceptualization of the clinical phenomenon as representing an intermediate state of personality organization between neurotic structures and psychotic decompensation. This structural model is seldom invoked in current discussions. Although patient groups, patient advocate groups, and some professionals have expressed dissatisfaction with this label, there has been no consensus on an alternative title in the professional literature. Some of the potential alternative labels we have heard are "emotionally unstable personality," "emotionally dysregulated personality," and "complex trauma personality disorder." There are conceptual and theoretical difficulties with all these alternative labels. In sum, it appears few like the current label, yet no one has come up with a more acceptable alternative. Unfortunately, this situation continues with DSM-5.

Histrionic Personality Disorder

DSM-5 offers no specific information on developmental issues in Histrionic Personality Disorder.

Narcissistic Personality Disorder

DSM-5 notes only that narcissistic traits are common during adolescence and do not predict the development of Narcissistic Personality Disorder. Although pathological narcissistic traits probably develop in childhood and adolescence, we have not found this to be a useful Personality Disorder diagnosis in youth. Noting apparently extreme narcissistic traits can be helpful in case conceptualization and management.

CLUSTER C (ANXIOUS–FEARFUL) PERSONALITY DISORDERS

Avoidant Personality Disorder

DSM-5 notes that shy and avoidant traits may be common in children and do not necessarily develop into Avoidant Personality Disorder. The available literature on avoidant personality problems suggests that these disorders usually do begin in childhood, when stranger shyness is common; however, in the typical developmental course, these excessive fear reactions decrease with social experience, whereas the problems increase with age and experience for the individual who will eventually be labeled as having Avoidant Personality Disorder. Sensitivity to this potential problem of youth is well advised, but caution seems prudent in applying a label of personality disorder to socially inhibited youth.

DSM-5 points out that Social Anxiety Disorder overlaps in symptomatic presentation with Avoidant Personality Disorder to a great extent. Indeed, these two categories may be two different conceptualizations of the same difficulty. Social Anxiety Disorder will often serve as an accurate diagnosis of a child who shows severe avoidant traits, and such a diagnosis will avoid the difficulties inherent in using Personality Disorder diagnoses with children.

Dependent Personality Disorder

DSM-5 also recommends great caution in the use of the Dependent Personality Disorder category with children and adolescents because a dependent pattern is developmentally typical and appropriate. If the presenting problems involve functioning apart from the caretaker, the category of Separation Anxiety Disorder should be considered. In our clinical work, we have noted dependent traits in children and adolescents but have never used this Personality Disorder diagnosis with youth.

Obsessive–Compulsive Personality Disorder

DSM-5 offers no information regarding the use of the Obsessive–Compulsive Personality Disorder category with children and adolescents. We have encountered no clinical cases of its use in our professional practice. A common mistake is the confusion of Obsessive–Compulsive Personality Disorder with Obsessive–Compulsive Disorder. The latter category involves specific symptoms (obsessions or compulsions), whereas the Personality Disorder pattern is a "preoccupation with orderliness, perfectionism, and mental and interpersonal control, at the expense of flexibility, openness, and efficiency" (p. 678). Despite the common elements in their labels (reflecting a previous belief in common psychodynamic features), the available evidence does not suggest an empirical linkage of these two problems. Adults with Obsessive–Compulsive Personality Disorder do not seem especially prone to manifest Obsessive–Compulsive Disorders as well; nor is Obsessive–Compulsive Personality Disorder commonly reported in individuals who present with Obsessive–Compulsive Disorder, although these two diagnoses have been reported to be comorbid in some clinical cases.

RESIDUAL CASES

Two options are provided for cases that meet the General Personality Disorder criteria (pp. 646–647) but do not meet the criteria for one of the specific DSM-5 categorical diagnoses. These options differ in whether the clinician indicates the specific reason that the client fails to meet criteria for a specific personality disorder. As in other areas, a diagnosis of Other Specified Personality Disorder would include the specifics regarding the case. The example in the text is: "e.g., 'mixed personality features'" (p. 684). The Unspecified Personality Disorder diagnosis is used when the examiner does not indicate why criteria for a specific personality disorder are not reached. The text gives the example of cases in which there is insufficient information to make a more specific diagnosis or the author chooses to not share the information. In our opinion, a good clinical report includes such discussion, so the Unspecified Personality Disorder category would hopefully be a rare creature.

ALTERNATIVE DSM-5 MODEL FOR PERSONALITY DISORDERS

Included in Section III of DSM-5, Emerging Measures and Models, is an alternative classification of personality disorders based on a dimensional model of personality functioning but leading to six personality disorder diagnoses plus a seventh category of Personality Disorder—Trait Specified to cover cases in which a personality disorder is judged to be present but the criteria for one of the six specific categories are not met. The approach considers level of personality functioning, the presence of pathological personality traits, and the pervasiveness and stability of traits and impairment. The personality trait model is roughly consistent with the five-factor model of personality. This model attempts to combine the literature of the past on personality disorders with one general model of personality theory. The text discusses the decision of the American Psychiatric Association Board of Trustees to retain the previous categorical model in Section II and include the new proposed model in Section III.

The alternative personality disorder section may have some advantages over the traditional personality disorder model. How useful in clinical practice and how much acceptance it can achieve among practitioners and researchers remains to be seen. It does not really address any of our fundamental concerns about making personality disorder diagnoses in children and adolescents. Personality disorders may well be a valid and useful way of thinking about individuals whose personality traits are so rigid, extreme, and enduring that these traits prove maladaptive in a wide range of the situations and persist over much of their lifespans. Individual differences in personality (whether viewed as fundamentally biological or learned or an interaction of biology and experience) arise early in life. Children show individual differences in their adaptability to experiences, and they carry the influence of these life experiences into subsequent experiences. That said, it is questionable how much confidence we can place in making personality disorder diagnoses in children or adolescents who are still going through fundamental periods of growth and development.

By most definitions in general and by the DSM definition in particular, personality disorders are enduring and cross-situational. How long is enduring? The manual suggests at least a year (p. 647), but this criterion seems to us totally inadequate in deciding to apply such a serious label that may well follow the individual throughout life. How pervasive must the maladaptive pattern be? The manual speaks of a "wide range of social and personal contexts" (p. 647) and a "broad range of social and personal situations" (p. 647), but how wide and broad a range of social and personal situations have children or adolescents experienced? Children and, to a lesser degree, adolescents are dependent upon their families, communities, and schools for their situational experiences. What appears consistently maladaptive within the narrow confines of a youth's world may seem less so when he or she achieves greater autonomy in building his or her social world and environment.

We find it useful clinically to attend to individual differences in ability and personality characteristics when evaluating children and adolescents. To discuss characteristics that are extreme, dysfunctional in common settings such as classrooms or neighborhoods, and persistent in the face of negative consequences is invaluable in a comprehensive evaluation of a youth. To make the inferential leap to a conclusion that these traits will endure and affect the child in environments in which they as yet have had no experiences seems seldom to be justified. In short, we find that personality disorder diagnoses contribute little to our work with youth, either for assessment or treatment.

16

Additional Codes and Categories

OTHER MENTAL DISORDERS

DSM-5 tries to preserve some of the breadth and flexibility introduced in DSM-IV classifications while simultaneously aiming to reduce the (possible) overreliance on residual case diagnoses (i.e., the previous "Not Otherwise Specified" diagnoses). In addition to the domain-specific Other Specified and Unspecified categories, there are four broadband diagnoses that offer additional coverage of the potential mental health concerns observed by examiners. They are Other Specified Mental Disorder Due to Another Medical Condition, Unspecified Mental Disorder Due to Another Medical Condition, Other Specified Mental Disorder, and Unspecified Mental Disorder. All four diagnoses are Mental Disorders; that is, the examiner's conclusion in using one of these diagnoses is that a case meets the basic definition of a Mental Disorder within DSM-5. However, the examiner's conclusion is also either that the case does not meet the criteria for a diagnosis in any of the more focused areas of problem behavior or that inadequate information is available to indicate whether the case does meet criteria for a more specific category. Again, the difference between "Other Specified" and "Unspecified" is whether the examiner chooses to communicate the reason the presentation does not meet criteria for a more specific diagnosis ("Other Specified") or opts not to provide this information ("Unspecified"). The text suggests that the designation of Unspecified may be more likely in some settings, such as brief encounters in emergency rooms. That said, indicating the basis upon which a diagnosis was made, even if it is only to note that insufficient information was available at that time, is good clinical practice. From this consideration, it is likely that most indeterminate cases would be classified as Other Specified.

Two diagnoses that are interestingly missing from DSM-5 are DSM-IV-TR diagnoses of V71.09 No Diagnosis or Condition (which was used on both Axis I or Axis II) and 799.9 Diagnosis Deferred (which was also available for use on Axis I or II). The No Diagnosis category was an affirmative statement. That is, the school psychologist had evaluated a young person and his or her situation and had concluded that a Mental Disorder was not present. There may be problems in the young person's life or with his or her behavior, but these problems fall short of the definition of a Mental Disorder. In contrast, the Diagnosis Deferred category was a statement of doubt. That is, the examiner was unwilling to draw a firm conclusion about the (absence or) presence of a Mental Disorder. Such a diagnosis was not an answer; it was a statement that more time was needed to gather data so that a firmer conclusion could be drawn. It is not clear why these options do not appear in DSM-5.

OTHER CONDITIONS THAT MAY BE THE FOCUS OF CLINICAL ATTENTION

An extremely important section of DSM-5 is the chapter on "Other Conditions That May Be a Focus of Clinical Attention." This chapter covers problems and challenges that may significantly affect a child's adjustment and functioning but that are not deemed "Mental Disorders" within the framework of DSM. Recall that DSM follows a medical model in which the focus is on the individual: A Mental Disorder is a description of a condition experienced and manifested by an individual. Relational or situational issues, such as child abuse or poverty, are known to be tremendously important factors and may need therapeutic attention, but these are not Mental Disorders. This section of the text identifies many of these "other conditions" and provides the relevant ICD codes. Parenthetically, it is worth knowing that historically most of these conditions in ICD-9-CM were identified with an alphanumeric designation beginning with the letter "V," as opposed to the disorders in ICD-9-CM, which were all numerical. These "other conditions" were often colloquially referred to as the "V codes." In ICD-10, which moves to an alphanumeric system for all codes, these other conditions begin with the letter Z.

For psychologists and other mental health practitioners working with youth, the importance of the Other Conditions section can hardly be overemphasized. These are the conditions that shape, for better or worse, many of the experiences that affect the child's behavior. Conflict in the family system, education and (for some teenagers) occupational difficulties, and maltreatment in all its forms are well-known environmental influences on adjustment, self-esteem, and interpersonal functioning. Other situational issues, such as poverty, homelessness, and discrimination or persecution, blight the lives of far too many youth. Challenges from unplanned pregnancies, exposure to terrorism or war, and involvement with the legal system as victim or perpetrator are, unfortunately, not unknown to some youth. DSM-5 is to be complimented in providing a much more extensive selection of the Other Conditions codes available in ICD-9-CM and ICD-10. This expanded coverage may reflect, in part, the move away from the previous multiaxial system, in which, with or without ICD coding, many of these factors were discussed on Axis IV: Psychosocial and Environmental Problems.

A few available conditions/codes within this chapter deserve particular attention. For example, the Borderline Intellectual Functioning code continues from DSM-IV-TR as a designation for those cases in which a youth's mental ability does not fall within the criteria of Intellectual Disability but is the focus of clinical attention or is seen as a significant influence in the youth's adjustment, response to treatment, or prognosis. Approximately 6% of the general population has IQs between 70 and 79. Most of these individuals would not meet criteria in DSM-5 as having an Intellectual Disability, yet their educational successes and failures, their occupational futures, their capacities to adapt to environmental challenges, and their coping mechanisms may be significantly affected by their lower cognitive abilities. They may be at greater risk to develop mental disorders, and their adjustment may be greatly enhanced by appropriate support and, if needed, counseling. As with other conditions, the availability of a formal designation and code (V62.89 in ICD-9-CM or R41.83 in ICD-10) can provide documentation of need, access to services, and a basis for further research into developmental risks and empirically supported educational interventions.

The Child or Adolescent Antisocial Behavior (V71.02/Z72.810) category addresses cases of severe misbehavior or criminal activity in a youth that does not meet criteria for a mental disorder, such as Conduct Disorder or Intermittent Explosive Disorder. Many of the youth who move through our juvenile justice system do not have Mental Disorders (and many do that are often unrecognized, but that is another issue and challenge), but they are engaging in dangerous and/or illegal behavior that can have serious life consequences. An interesting paradox here is that the title of the category often sounds to many novice professionals as more damning than an actual Mental Disorder such as Conduct Disorder. Nevertheless, this designation often has less ominous prognostic implications than Conduct Disorder. Much of the broader sociological and psychological literature on delinquency would be captured by this category.

Acculturation Difficulty (V62.4/Z60.3) addresses the adjustment difficulties attendant upon moving into a new culture. Continuing issues surrounding migration into the United States and acculturation to a new home and circumstances are particularly common in some areas of the nation, but they may present to any mental health professional in almost any locale. Similarly, the enhanced perception of the deleterious effects of bullying in youth give an especial appreciation of the availability of a clear designation of this problem in the category Social Exclusion or Rejection (V62.4/Z60.4) and Target of (Perceived) Adverse Discrimination or Persecution (V62.4/Z60.5). The reader will note the enhanced specificity of ICD-10 over ICD-9-CM with these two codes.

In addition to codes to document exposure to poverty and low income and other adverse environmental circumstances, DSM-5 has two codes to identify lack of appropriate treatment resources: Unavailability or Inaccessibility of Health Care Facilities and Unavailability or Inaccessibility of Other Helping Agencies. Even with all the efforts of the past few years, a disturbing number of youth live in families lacking access to basic medical and other health care services. With respect to the psychological adjustment of youth, a conundrum of the increasing development of empirically supported treatments for behavioral and emotional problems is that trained practitioners or agencies supporting these specialized treatments are often not available within a community. Thus, these codes are by no means anything approaching an answer, but at least the potential to document such problems is a first step toward a solution.

Two other categories that deserve the reader's attention in this group are Nonadherence to Medical Treatment (V15.81/Z91.19) and Malingering (V65.2/Z76.5). Treatment noncompliance can be an issue with any population but sometimes is a critical issue with youth, most of whom do not seek treatment on their own. A fundamental difference in mental health questions regarding youth and adults is that, relative to adults who seek out mental health services on their own initiative, most children are brought into mental health facilities by adult caretakers because of concerns the adults have. This referral difference plays out in many different ways and is one factor dramatically affecting the prevalence differences often reported between the general population and the clinical population. A foundational aspect of mental health services is building a working relationship that allows the client to participate in helpful activities, even when these may be stressful or unfamiliar or seemingly strange ways to act. Although a noncompliance category has the potential to be nothing more than "blaming the victim" for our failure to forge such a therapeutic relationship, it can provide a means to spotlight the nature of the difficulty.

In contrast to deliberate noncooperation with treatment, Malingering refers to the deliberate production or assumption of symptoms to generate the impression of illness for some external gain. Three DSM categories focus on instances in which an apparent problem is not the real problem: Conversion Disorder, Factitious Disorder, and Malingering. In each case we see symptoms that, in some sense, are not "real." The differences between these three diagnoses lie in (1) whether the symptoms are being deliberately, intentionally, or willfully produced by the client and (2) whether there is a clear external motivation for the symptom production. In a Conversion Disorder, the symptoms of an apparent physical, sensory, or neurological deficit are not the result of any medical injury, illness, or traditional neurological condition, yet the client is not "putting on." That is, he or she is not faking. The client's perception is that of a genuine experience of the weakness, blindness, or convulsions as reported. Although there may be external, secondary gain, the motivations for conversion symptoms are not usually primary maintaining contingencies. In Malingering the individual is "faking it." The individual is aware that he or she is deliberately feigning the symptoms seen, and the individual is feigning the symptoms for a clear motivation, such as receiving disability compensation, avoiding work, or getting to stay home from school. In Factitious Disorder, the individual is also intentionally dissimulating, but the motivation seems to be only to assume the special status of being a patient, being ill, or having a condition. Malingering, in its milder and temporary manifestations, is probably quite common in youth, but clinical cases are rare. So too are Conversion Disorder and Factitious Disorders in youth. Factitious Disorder by Proxy, a disorder in which an adult produces symptoms in his or her child in order to obtain "parent of a sick child" status, would likely constitute child maltreatment and would receive the appropriate DSM-5 classification from the Other Conditions grouping.

These are only a few of the available categories in this section of DSM-5. Careful reading and consideration of this chapter will greatly enhance the professional's capacity to identify and document the multiple aspects of a youth's situation, challenges, and adjustment.

EMERGING MEASURES AND MODELS

A final set of diagnostic categories the school psychologist needs to be aware of is found in Section III of DSM-5, Emerging Measures and Models. In this section are proposed categories, alternative theoretical models, and other functional assessments that were judged to have sufficient merit to warrant investigation but were not deemed ready for inclusion in the main text of DSM-5. A few of these categories have already been discussed earlier in this book. In almost every case for which one of these specific diagnostic categories might be used, the diagnosis should be formally coded as an Other Specified category in the appropriate DSM grouping. The provision of criterion sets for these patterns should help stimulate research and generate a database that will support (or reject) their inclusion in future versions of DSM-5 (DSM-5.2, etc.) or DSM-6.

A number of assessment measures are discussed in Section III, including the Cross-Cutting Symptom Measures, the Clinician-Rated Dimensions of Psychosis Severity, and the World Health Organization Disability Assessment Schedule (WHODAS 2.0; Üstün et al., 2010). The issue of cultural formulation is given much greater attention than in previous versions of the DSM, and a Cultural Formulation Interview is reviewed. The issue of dimensional assessment of personality disorders is addressed. These inclusions are potentially helpful and powerful additions to the DSM. It will be interesting to see the degree to which these approaches to assessment begin to influence clinical practice and documentation. For adult clients, the WHODAS 2.0 is viewed as a superior replacement for the Axis V Global Assessment of Functioning (GAF) rating that was made by clinicians in DSM-III through DSM-IV-TR. One version of the WHODAS is a client self-report device that is available in several forms. "Other"-rated and therapist-rated versions of the WHODAS are also available, but training is recommended before clinicians use that adaptation. The WHODAS has the advantage of being freely available and supported by a good deal of research (Üstün et al., 2010). How commonly it will actually be used remains to be seen. Another issue is the need for a child and adolescent version of the WHODAS. A youth version of the WHODAS is not yet available, but the World Health Organization has one in development. It would be helpful to have both an adolescent self-report measure and a parent/other adult informant version to aid in the assessment and diagnosis of youth.

The Section III chapter "Conditions for Further Study" includes research criterion sets for eight proposed diagnostic categories: Attenuated Psychosis Syndrome, Depressive Episodes With Short-Duration Hypomania, Persistent Complex Bereavement Disorder, Caffeine Use Disorder, Internet Gaming Disorder, Neurobehavioral Disorder Associated With Prenatal Alcohol Exposure, Suicidal Behavior Disorder, and Nonsuicidal Self-Injury. The last four have clear potential applicability to youth. Internet Gaming Disorder would presumably join Gambling Disorder in the substance abuse and addictive behavior disorder grouping. Neurobehavioral Disorder Associated With Prenatal Alcohol Exposure is intended to bring greater clarity to the behavioral consequences of fetal alcohol syndrome.

The final two potential diagnoses would provide classification of a major area of concern in mental health: suicidal behavior and deliberate self-injury. Without addressing the merits or limitations of any of these proposed categories, we simply note that these are not currently diagnoses available in the DSM-5 system. How the behaviors would be dealt with within current DSM-5 categories is unclear in the text. Suicidal and parasuicidal behavior could be symptoms of a number of DSM-5 diagnoses, most of which would have an Other Specified option if full criteria for a specific diagnosis were not met. An Unspecified Neurocognitive Disorder option seems to be a possible current classification of Neurobehavioral Disorder Associated With Prenatal Alcohol Exposure. It is not clear how self-defeating Internet gaming behavior would be dealt with in the available diagnoses.

Part III

THE APPLICATION OF DSM-5 IN SCHOOL SETTINGS

Issues and Topics

In teaching psychological evaluation courses to graduate students, we have found that one of the most important tasks has been helping students understand the difference between psychological testing and psychological assessment. Testing is an essentially mechanical process that can be taught with relative ease and simplicity. Even the most challenging of psychological tests—from the perspective of the tasks required of the examiner—could be taught adequately to high school graduates with average intelligence. Psychological assessment, in contrast, is a highly demanding, professional-level task requiring an understanding of human problems, awareness of issues in accurate testing, knowledge of the characteristics of available approaches to evaluation and characteristics of available instruments, and the integration of all this understanding and knowledge in the individual case to generate an evaluation approach that can answer the referral questions. It follows from this logic that psychiatric classification involves more than memorizing a set of diagnostic criteria. In most cases, we discourage students from even trying to memorize the DSM criterion sets. What evaluators need is an understanding of the process of human evaluation, thorough familiarity with (though not rote knowledge of) the classification system to be used, and a thoughtful selection of the most appropriate diagnostic codes. Like most other human activity, the process of psychiatric classification interacts with many other systems of behavior, codes of ethics and values, and people. In this final section, several topics related to the competent and professional use of DSM-5 in the classification of emotional and behavioral problems in youth are considered.

17

Ethics and Professional Responsibility in Evaluation

THE ROLE OF THE SCHOOL PSYCHOLOGIST IN MENTAL HEALTH ASSESSMENT

The issue of which professions should be involved in making emotional and behavioral classifications is a complicated one, probably with both rational and less than rational elements. There is a lack of consensus even over what the activity should be called: "psychiatric diagnosis," "mental health assessment," "behavioral diagnosis," or the like. Professional pride and vanity, legal definitions of medical and psychological practice, discipline/guild issues of professional autonomy and economic competition, and the social forces that have shaped and reshaped mental health practice in the 20th and early 21st centuries have all played a role. The broad topic of psychology as an independent profession is well beyond the scope of this book, but the specific question of what role school psychologists should play in behavioral classification is important.

Psychologists have long been involved in the classification of behavioral and emotional disorders. One obvious area of this involvement has been psychological testing within mental health services. Testing was for a long period the special province of psychologists, and to the degree that testing proved valuable to the process of evaluation, psychologists were drawn into this process (despite any contrary opinions). For the intellectual, academic, and cognitive disorders, the role of formal psychometric assessment is often primary. Few professionals of any discipline would attempt to diagnose intellectual disability, learning disabilities, or dementia without formal ability testing. The contributions of behavior rating scales to the evaluation of many childhood problems, of symptom report scales to the assessment of mood and anxiety problems, and of global measures of temperament and social relationships to models of personality dysfunction are all well documented. One could well argue that the extensive preparation in assessment that is a part of most psychology training programs places psychologists in an optimal position for making reliable and valid assessments of patterns of maladjustment. Clinical and counseling psychologists in a wide range of professional settings are routinely called upon to make classifications of their clients within the format of DSM-5.

School psychologists have been no less involved in the assessment and description of behavior and behavior problems than psychologists in other applied specialties have been. Their work traditions, however, have often not involved expressing these evaluations in the language of a psychiatric classification system, at least when they are practicing in schools. The highly competent assessments of school psychologists have usually been aimed at establishing young persons' eligibility for special services within the educational system, helping to plan individualized education programs (IEPs), or monitoring change and progress over the course of young people's educational careers. Even the first of these functions has generally been carried out in the context of a quite different and specialized classification system, developed within and largely restricted to school settings and educational purposes. The psychological assessments of most school psychologists have contained data based on behavioral observations, psychological testing, historical records, and the report of significant others in a child's or adolescent's life but have not usually contained any expression of how this information would be represented within the DSM-5 classification system. Until recently, this has not been viewed as essential in the role of the school psychologist.

Numerous influences, however, have begun to change this state of affairs. School psychologists and the educational systems that employ them are increasingly asking whether psychiatric classification should be part of the school psychologist's role. One obviously powerful factor is economics. Mental health diagnosis makes available the possibility of accessing other potential sources of funding for psychological services within schools—the "third-party payers" of insurance companies, as well as state and federal government agencies. With increasing legislative mandates to provide an ever-enlarging range of services, often without any corresponding additional funding, schools are being pressed to the limits of their financial resources. Some schools have begun exploring the possibility of accessing commercial insurance and Medicaid funding for psychological services directed at the mental health problems of children and adolescents. Access to these funds, however, almost always requires a DSM classification, and the person within a school system most qualified to deal with the issue of psychiatric classification is the school psychologist.

Based on our experiences in school, clinic, residential, and hospital settings, we have no hesitation in asserting that school psychologists are just as capable of making competent psychiatric classifications as their colleagues in clinical and counseling psychology. Understanding maladjustment is an essential task for all applied psychologists, and the DSM-5 classification system is an important tool in working with psychopathology. We contend that psychologists in all applied specialties need to develop and maintain a role in the ongoing development and application of this tool. To do otherwise is to risk becoming increasingly irrelevant in the field of mental health.

The application of professional psychology is a legally regulated activity in all states. State licensing laws differ in their recognition of formal psychiatric diagnosis as a role for the psychologist. Any psychologist considering expanding his or her professional role should seek appropriate training and supervision and should also carefully review any legal regulations pertaining to this potential area of new practice (see the following Professional Note). Consultation with an attorney who has expertise in mental health practice may well be advisable in such situations. These prudent cautions notwithstanding, developing expertise with using the DSM-5 classification system to codify the emotional and behavioral problems of children and adolescents is an appropriate professional activity for school psychologists. Furthermore, it is likely that such expertise will be increasingly called upon and that the use of DSM-5 will eventually become an essential activity of school psychologists, just as it currently is for clinical and counseling psychologists.

BEST-PRACTICE RECOMMENDATIONS FOR SCHOOL PSYCHOLOGISTS REGARDING DIAGNOSIS

No single activity alone is sufficient for the development of a new area of competence. The school psychologist wishing to develop novel skills in mental health diagnosis should proceed exactly the same way as in the development of any other new set of skills. Reading and study, continuing educational workshops, supervised practice, and frequent professional consultation throughout the early stages of independent practice are all part of the ongoing professional development of all psychologists. Providing documentation of one's preparation to engage in various aspects of professional psychology is a common expectation, and the school psychologist should do this just as carefully as he or she develops skills in mental health diagnosis. Everything from the casual inquiry of a straightforwardly curious colleague to the pointed examination of an attorney for whom a particular classification is not a welcome development can present the school psychologist with an opportunity to explain how he or she engages in mental health diagnosis and how he or she has prepared for this role.

Professional Note. Review of District Policies and State Regulations Regarding Mental Health Diagnosis

As a school psychologist or allied mental health professional prepares to confront the practical issues of psychiatric diagnosis, it is also prudent to review relevant agency guidelines and statutory regulation of this activity. School districts, special education units, and other employers may have formal or informal policies covering the use of behavioral classification. The professional action of diagnosing a mental disorder may be regulated or licensed by the state. Reviewing relevant policy and statutes, seeking input from professional associations, and consultation with more experienced peers can all serve to highlight potential problems, identify appropriate solutions, and reduce the anxiety commonly felt when one is moving into a new area of professional development. Some state associations for school psychologists have developed recommendations for seeking third-party reimbursement that address the issue of diagnosis (see, e.g., Elliott et al., 1993).

18

The Case Record

Data and Supporting Documentation for Diagnosis

The case record of a child or adolescent contains all the essential records and documentation necessary for the provision of psychological services. Part of this record should include the mental health classification made and any relevant data bearing on the issue of diagnosis. In many settings, applied psychologists are required to note after any diagnosis the data supporting this classification: for example, "Conduct Disorder as manifested by. . . . " It is a prudent habit to develop. In case notes, it is sound practice to list the signs and symptoms supporting any working or final diagnoses. The best way to defend any diagnostic statement made is to point out the behavioral phenomena that form the basis for the classification. Because mental health records may follow an individual for a long time, it is essential that sufficient documentation and data be maintained to allow a future review of any diagnosis.

CONFIDENTIALITY, FREEDOM OF INFORMATION, AND PARENTS' AND CHILDREN'S RIGHTS

An important topic to consider in the professional activity of any psychologist is maintaining the privacy and confidentiality of information about clients. In addition to the ethical requirements of the profession, there are specific legal requirements governing the protection and circumstances for legal release of psychological records in most states. If mental health classification becomes a part of a child's or adolescent's school records, it is advisable to determine whether additional legal requirements regarding confidentiality apply. The statutes governing mental health information may differ from those covering educational data. Mental health confidentiality laws can be complex, especially for adolescents, who may be treated as more autonomous than children but are not yet fully emancipated.

Schools are usually held responsible not only for withholding information without appropriate releases but also for providing information to parents or other legal guardians. This sharing of records typically includes mental health information. The practicing psychologist needs to be comfortable discussing a client's psychiatric diagnosis with a mature client or the parents of an immature client, or, in the case of a teenager, with both the adolescent and his or her parents. Again, it is important to be familiar with the specific legal mandates that apply to a particular state and with the policies and procedures of a particular work setting. With the issue of mental health classification, there may not be a policy in effect because such classification has not been a practice within that school system in the past. Developing a written policy may be one of the first tasks for the school psychologist who has moved into this area of practice.

It is good practice to maintain a record of any information disclosed from a case record. If the release is to be of copies of records, we recommend noting on the release-of-information form what documents were copied, to whom they were transmitted, and the date. If the release is oral, we recommend including a summary of the information discussed in the case notes.

MAINTENANCE OF RECORDS

Mental health records need to be maintained securely, both to protect client confidentiality and to provide for their legitimate release at a client's request. The importance of a longitudinal database seems undeniable in our attempts to understand human development, both adaptive and maladaptive, more clearly. The most solid basis for resolving difficult diagnostic questions is often found in the documentation of the course a young person's problem takes over time.

Providing for the secure storage and maintenance of records should not be a new responsibility for any school system. It may, however, be prudent to review state requirements for maintenance of records with respect to mental health records if DSM-5 diagnoses are being added to the case data generated within school records (see the following Professional Note).

As we have noted before, laws may be different for mental health records than they are for educational records. If DSM-5 diagnoses are included in a child's educational file, it is likely that these records will be considered mental health records by a court and that the applicable confidentiality acts will apply.

Professional Note. Maintenance of Mental Health Records

One variation of a common joke among psychologists and other mental health professionals is the following: "How long should mental health records be retained? Forever plus 7 years." Although there is no absolute answer to the question posed in this joke, it is an important practical issue for both the school psychologist and the school district. The relevant state statutes governing appropriate handling of mental health records may differ from those pertaining to educational records. In addition, the potential role mental health records may play if a question of professional malpractice or liability is ever raised is an important consideration. The school psychologist should carefully consider the issues regarding maintenance of mental health records, and the school district should develop a formal policy (if none exists). A review of documents such as the American Psychological Association's (2007) guidelines is a good starting point.

19

Seeking Reimbursement for Assessment and Diagnosis within School Settings

PHYSICIANS' *CURRENT PROCEDURAL TERMINOLOGY* CODES

The American Medical Association's *Current Procedural Terminology (CPT)* is a system used to identify medical procedures, including diagnostic procedures for mental health concerns. It was originally developed by the American Medical Association in 1966 as a means of reporting the services performed by physicians. The codes are now revised yearly and are available from the American Medical Association. The CPT gives descriptive phrases to identify professional activities and assigns a five-digit code to each one (e.g., psychological testing by a psychologist is coded 96101). It provides a uniform method of documenting health care activities and especially of communicating with third-party payers (i.e., insurance companies, state or federal government agencies). The 1983 update of CPT was adopted by the Health Care Financing Administration (HCFA) as part of that agency's common procedural coding system for reporting services to the Medicare and Medicaid programs, and subsequent revisions have continued to serve as the primary basis for accessing these potential sources of reimbursement (Schmidt, Yowell, & Jaffe, 2010). Most insurance companies require CPT codes to be used in all claims submitted. The school psychologist or school system seeking reimbursement from insurance companies or public programs will usually need to be able to document these claims in terms of these codes. Information is available through the

American Medical Association, the American Psychological Association, and other professional associations on the use of CPT codes. Most of the professional activity involved in psychological evaluation and diagnosis is reflected in the following CPT codes: 90101, Psychological testing, interpretation, and reporting per hour by a psychologist; 96102, Psychological test per hour by a technician; 96103, Psychological testing by a computer, including time for the psychologist's interpretation and reporting; 96111, Developmental Testing, Extended; 96116, Neurobehavioral Status Exam; 96118, Neuropsychological testing, interpretation, and reporting by a psychologist; 96119, Neuropsychological testing, interpretation, and reporting by a technician; 96120, Neuropsychological testing by a computer, including time for the psychologist's interpretation and reporting. Other codes are available for psychotherapy and other services.

Submission of claims to most third-party payers either requires or is greatly facilitated by the use of a standard health insurance claim form, usually identified as the HCFA-1500 form. This form (available from many companies providing business supplies for medical settings and physicians) provides a standardized format for the recording of information on the patient, his or her insurance, the medical procedures conducted, and their relation to diagnoses, as well as information on the provider of the services. As with any complex system, initial experiences with the HCFA-1500 can be quite frustrating; however, the range of potential psychological services and procedures is really quite limited, and billing for psychological evaluation can usually become the province of the technical support staff after some initial familiarity with the form has been gained. (Of course, regardless of who completes a form, the licensed psychologist who signs the form is responsible for the accuracy of the information contained and should carefully review any submission for reimbursement.)

"MEDICAL NECESSITY" AS A CRITERION

Commercial insurance companies and governmental insurance programs (e.g., Medicare, Medicaid, Social Security, Civilian Health and Medicaid Program of the Uniformed Services [CHAMPUS]) employ various controls and restrictions on reimbursement for medical services. Much of the attention is focused on the reimbursement of treatment, but evaluations will also fall under these guidelines if assessment services are covered by an insurance policy. Typically, the policy will indicate that only services that are "medically necessary," or some other phrase to this effect, will be considered for potential reimbursement. Some policies will reimburse for services only if a physician has made the referral. The third-party payer often makes the final determination of what is "medically necessary."

Some insurance companies, for instance, may not deem it appropriate to reimburse for psychological services to treat an adolescent with problems of isolated antisocial behavior (V71.02 [Z72.810], Child or Adolescent Antisocial Behavior—an "Other Conditions That May Be a Focus of Clinical Attention" classification) because this designation is not a Mental Disorder. The same insurance company may help pay for the exact same services in another young person if the diagnosis is 312.32 [F91.2], Conduct Disorder, Adolescent-Onset Type, or 309.3 [F43.24], Adjustment Disorder With Disturbance of Conduct.

These differing determinations can be frustrating for the psychologist because the exact same psychological services may be provided in both cases; however, the decision does make sense from the perspective of the insurance company. In the second case, the problem is identified as a Mental Disorder. The holder of the insurance policy has paid for coverage of Mental Disorders, and it is the obligation of the insurance company to provide this coverage. Note that the insurance company does not have an obligation either to provide unlimited help to the policy holder or to support the psychologist providing the services in "doing good." The obligations of the insurer to the insured are explicitly laid out in the insurance policy. Despite frequent advertisement themes suggesting that insurance companies are policyholders' friends and will watch out for them, the actual relationship is carefully governed by contract and law. It is prudent to remember that to reimburse a claim not covered under a holder's contract would be an unethical act for the insurance company. Such behavior would reduce the legitimate profits of the shareholders of the company and could ultimately lead to rate increases for all policyholders.

With respect to determining psychiatric diagnoses, assessment and evaluation services may often be more broadly covered under a mental health policy than treatment services may be. For instance, in some cases the evaluation of a potential mental disorder may be determined to be eligible for reimbursement, even if the condition that is ultimately diagnosed is one that is not eligible for coverage. As long as an eligible condition is being actively considered in the evaluation process (i.e., being "ruled out"), this process itself may be eligible. Individual policies vary widely, however, and it is never safe to rely on generalizations about psychological conditions, services, or insurance companies. What matters is the exact insurance contract that the client has purchased with the third-party carrier or the contract that has been negotiated by the client's employer.

Potential insurance reimbursement for any psychological service will depend on the exact nature of coverage for mental health services in the insured's policy. Most policies covering mental health services have "deductibles" that must be satisfied prior to recovery of any funds; will typically reimburse only a portion of "the usual and customary fees" for a service in that area; and/or may have yearly or lifetime "caps" for a particular disorder, which set an upper limit on the amount of potential total reimbursement. A good deal of unhappiness can be avoided by carefully and accurately determining how services will be paid for before these services are provided. Clients often overestimate how helpful their health insurance policies will be in supporting mental health services. Although dated, Small's (1991) text is one of the few published references on this topic. Online resources provided by professional associations may be the most helpful, current resources on this topic.

ETHICAL AND PROFESSIONAL RESPONSIBILITIES IN BILLING

School psychologists usually have a great deal of experience in carrying out psychological evaluations. The output of these evaluations may not have been expressed in the language of DSM-5, but the process of careful and accurate assessment has been well developed in every competently trained school psychologist. Applying these skills to the use of the DSM-5 classification system is a minor extension. School psychologists, usually by both natural inclination and formal training, also have a mental set to be helpful to their clients. They are motivated to provide as much assistance as possible to young people, their teachers, and their parents and families. However, school psychologists usually have not had much experience in billing for psychological services and in interacting with insurance companies or other third-party carriers. This lack of exposure creates the potential for some difficulties.

School psychologists who are moving into the role of seeking reimbursement for psychological services need to think carefully through their professional role and responsibilities. The job of a school psychologist carrying out a psychological evaluation is to make the best assessment of the young person and of his or her situation that is possible under the circumstances. The job of such a psychologist who makes use of the DSM-5 classification system is to express the results in the most appropriate DSM-5 code or codes—to choose the DSM-5 category or categories that most accurately and validly capture the essential features of the youth's situation. The job of the school psychologist is *not* to help the school system or the young person's parents obtain insurance reimbursement for the care given in the case. At least, it is not directly the responsibility of the school psychologist to do anything and everything possible to achieve reimbursement.

Certainly the psychologist should be willing to provide records (with appropriately executed releases of information) to support insurance claims. The school system may file the claims, and it may even be part of the psychologist's job to file the claims (not an efficient use of professional time, though it does happen). But the issue of potential reimbursement must not enter into any decision about classification. Diagnostic decision making cannot be influenced by what may happen when the case is reviewed by an insurance company for possible reimbursement under a medical insurance policy. Reimbursement decisions have no place in decisions about diagnosis. If these considerations are given a place in diagnostic classification, the basic validity of the process is violated. The integrity of the evaluation has been lost. To base a diagnosis on anything other than the behavioral facts of the case is unethical. If such a diagnosis is used to try to obtain reimbursement, it is usually illegal because it is considered an act of fraud against the insurance company or other third-party payer.

Graduate students in diagnostic classes are anxious about making mistakes. They are concerned over disagreements regarding diagnosis. They want to be sure that their diagnoses are correct. Although such concerns are understandable and reasonable up to a point, the reality is that each diagnosis of human behavior is at best a calculated hypothesis based on the data known at that time. Subsequently acquired information may require a change in the diagnosis. This update does not mean that the first diagnosis was wrong and the second is right; both were based on the data available at the time of diagnosis. As we have repeatedly pointed out in this book, clinical judgment continues to play the decisive role in the DSM-5 classification system. Clinical judgment is the interpretation of the available data by the diagnosing professional; it is the weighing of various bits of information that support the diagnosis offered. A great deal of effort has gone into making the DSM-5 criteria as objective as possible, but there is still a great deal of room for honest differences of opinion. Two examiners may legitimately reach different final classifications of an individual case. Although we should strive to resolve such differences whenever possible, their occurrence cannot be eliminated from the application of DSM-5.

Neither the profession nor society at large expects perfect agreement; however, psychologists are expected to operate within the rules. The ultimate rule for proper psychiatric diagnosis is that classification needs to be based on the behavioral data available for each case. A psychologist who has proceeded on this basis will be able to show the data to justify a particular classification. Even if it is later determined that this diagnosis is not correct, there is little risk for either the psychologist or his or her agency if he or she acts in good faith. Again, society does not expect psychologists to be perfect, but it does expect psychologists to operate within their own rules. If a diagnosis is based on any consideration other than the known facts of the case, then a psychologist does assume a great risk, both personally and for the public status and reputation of psychology.

A full discussion of the practicalities of billing for mental health services and attending to relevant legal and ethical concerns is beyond the scope of this book, but readers are advised to explore these topics in detail. A good starting point is the online resources provided by professional organizations such as the American Psychological Association, the National Association of School Psychologists, and the American Counseling Association. Each of these organizations provides materials (for members only) to assist in executing these aspects of professional practice.

DIAGNOSTIC DISAGREEMENT

A related issue concerns agreement among diagnosticians. One driving force behind the wholesale changes introduced in DSM-III, which has continued to reverberate in the subsequent revisions, was the need for better reliability in psychiatric diagnosis. As differential treatments began to become available for a number of psychiatric disorders, a need for treatment evaluation research developed. Such research, however, required a reliable and valid classification system to establish treatment and control groups. There was general recognition of the unreliability of DSM-II, and without adequate reliability, validity was a moot concern. The objectivity, explicit criterion sets, and diagnostic decision rules of DSM-III, DSM-III-R, DSM-IV, DSM-IV-TR, and DSM-5 were intended to increase the reliability to an acceptable level. A review of the field study data suggests that considerable progress has been made toward this end. Given access to the same data, different evaluators are probably more likely to arrive at the same or related diagnoses with DSM-5 than with any previous classification tool.

"Given access to the same data," however, is the key phrase in the preceding sentence. Mental health professionals do not always have the same information with which to work. Developing skills in eliciting diagnostic data efficiently and comprehensively is a major career task for professionals from diverse disciplines. The task of obtaining the necessary data to arrive at DSM-5 diagnoses is beyond the intention or capacity of this book, but other references do address this important topic (Kronenberger & Meyer, 2001; Meyer & Weaver, 2006). One clear advantage of DSM-5 is a relatively clear formulation of what types of information are helpful and necessary to establish, support, and document a diagnostic formulation.

The task of the evaluator is always to make the best, most accurate classification based on the specific data available for a child or adolescent at the time. It needs to be emphasized that this formulation will not always agree with previous or future assessments by different mental health professionals, or even by the same professional. If a diagnosis is based on the best formulation of all of the data that are available at that time, it is the correct diagnosis. Other professionals may have the benefit of additional historical facts, collateral reports, clinical observations, reports of responses to treatment efforts, and/or further course data. Based in part on all of these data, new formulations of the young person's difficulties may be generated. This situation does not mean that the original diagnosis was wrong or incorrect. Again, if the diagnosis was based fairly on the known information at that time, then it was the correct diagnosis. A revision of a diagnostic formulation does not imply an error on anyone's part. Neither does a difference of opinion between two professionals involved in a child's or adolescent's care. As has been previously noted, DSM-5 provides substantial opportunities for clinical judgment, differential evaluation of the functional significance of symptomatic behavior, and attention to idiosyncratic features of a case to influence case formulations. However, this flexibility comes at a cost: Different mental health professionals will not always see a young person's case as best formulated in the same way. The DSM system does provide a framework that can be used for an objective review of diagnostic differences, but these differences will not always be completely resolved.

To reiterate once more, the school psychologist's job is to evaluate a child's or adolescent's emotional and behavioral problems in a fair, objective, and comprehensive manner and to base his or her diagnostic formulation on the facts that are currently available, not on concerns about reimbursement or on any other considerations. If another professional arrives at a different diagnosis, it may be interesting and worthy of discussion, but it does not necessarily have any implications for the psychologist's work. All professionals need to be willing to consider new information as it becomes available. A diagnosis may be revised in the light of new data, but this openness to revision does not mean that the previous classification was in error. It may have been completely accurate based on the understanding then available of the young person and his or her situation.

20

DSM-5 and the Individuals with Disabilities Education Improvement Act

Specific comparisons between the classifications of DSM-5 and those of the 2004 IDEA and its related 2006 regulations have been made in the IDEA Notes throughout Part II of this book. From a more general perspective, perhaps the most important consideration for the school psychologist or other child care professional is to recognize that, despite clear commonalities, the DSM-5 and IDEA systems constitute two distinctly different perspectives on children's adjustment problems. DSM-5 and IDEA both classify patterns of behavior shown by youth, and they are both categorical in their approach to classification. Both have a primary application in the allocation of resources (special services, treatments, medications, placement dispositions) for children and adolescents. Both are carefully constructed human documents, in which classifications have been arrived at through consideration of divergent viewpoints, empirical data, debate, and compromise. However, beyond these important similarities are major differences in coverage, focus, methodology, and purpose, which result in two qualitatively different taxonomies of behavior. These important differences make direct translation between DSM-5 and IDEA challenging. Relative to its predecessor, the diagnostic categories of DSM-5 do a much better job of aligning with IDEA classification categories, but they still do not perfectly map onto any simple set or subset of IDEA categories, even when there are major overlaps of clinical elements (e.g., autism, learning disability, and intellectual disability).

The coverage of DSM-5 is broad by intention; it attempts to classify all significant problems of behavior and adjustment across the lifespan. Some critics of the significant conceptual and methodological changes that occurred with DSM-III raised concern that the DSM system had become too inclusive—that issues of life adjustment and minor problems of common human experience had been recast as "mental disorders" to expand the domain of psychiatry or medicine. Even if this concern is set aside, everyone would agree that the intended coverage of DSM-5 is vastly greater than the range focused on by IDEA. A significant number of the Mental Disorders detailed in DSM-5 are irrelevant for the purposes of IDEA. DSM-5 focuses on identifying problematic patterns of behavior that cause great personal suffering or obvious impairment in life adaptation (Mental Disorders) or that are judged to be appropriate objects of therapeutic treatment or other intervention (V codes). By contrast, IDEA focuses on identifying psychological or medical disabilities that would prevent a child or adolescent from benefiting from public education unless appropriate remediation is made. It appears that many (but not all) DSM-5 Mental Disorders and some V codes affecting children and adolescents fall within the conceptualization of disability under IDEA; however, the correspondence is not perfect and often depends on features other than a diagnosis per se (e.g., the particular manifestations of the mental disorder or condition, the settings affected, and the influence on global adjustment or educational functioning).

The methodology of DSM-5 establishes objective criteria for the documentation of a Mental Disorder, but, with a few important exceptions, the methods of obtaining data relevant to these symptomatic criteria are left up to the examiner. The role of clinical judgment is extremely important, as is consistent with the origins of DSM-5 within the discipline of clinical medicine. The exact criteria used for the categories of IDEA are left to an important degree up to individual states and even to individual school districts. The methods of data collection, analysis, and determination of data quality and acceptability, however, are spelled out in IDEA and its revisions: nondiscriminatory and multidisciplinary assessment, parental involvement, and individualized education programs (IEPs). These important functional differences derive from the different purposes of these two efforts. DSM-5 is ultimately aimed at reliable and valid classification for the purposes of clinical treatment and research to improve clinical treatment. IDEA is ultimately aimed at providing safeguards so that all U.S. children have a fair and equal opportunity to benefit from public education. These are both important and laudable goals, but they are different; thus, the products of these two efforts are different, even when they sound alike (e.g., "intellectual disability" in IDEA and Intellectual Disability in DSM-5).

The definition of "behavioral disorders" offered within the IDEA legislation has itself been criticized on a number of grounds (Cline, 1990;

Council for Children with Behavioral Disorders, 1987), and alternative definitions have been proposed (Forness & Knitzer, 1990). Even within the federal government, there is incongruity between different definitions of "emotional disturbance" (Substance Abuse and Mental Health Services Administration, 2015). These definitions will be a subject of continuing discussion and debate as the United States struggles to accommodate the various educational, economic, political, medical, social, and psychological needs and realities that affect children's learning and development. Documentation of a DSM-5 Mental Disorder will often, perhaps usually, have relevance for a potential classification of a child or adolescent as eligible for special education or other special services under IDEA. The information involved in a DSM-5 diagnosis (symptoms, severity, course, effects, prognosis) will almost always be relevant, either positively or negatively, to establishment of eligibility under IDEA. Yet the categories of DSM-5 are not identical to those of IDEA. Some of the differences are perhaps minor ones in boundaries (e.g., age or degree of intellectual disability), in formulations (the molar categories of IDEA vs. the molecular categories of DSM-5), or in exact labels. The fundamental reality, however, is that some children with a DSM-5 diagnosis of a Mental Disorder are not deemed eligible for services under IDEA and some children who are eligible for services under IDEA do not have a Mental Disorder as defined by DSM-5. These are related but separate classification questions. The school psychologist may play a vital role in each determination, but each type of inquiry asks a unique question and deserves its own unique answer.

21

Concerns about DSM-5

This book has not addressed the various pros and cons of psychiatric classification. These advantages and disadvantages have been argued repeatedly, and there is good reason to continue considering the issue. No one who has walked the halls of a school for any length of time can really question the assertion that words can hurt, labels (informal or formal) can be hurled as weapons, and the emotional pain that can result is just as palpable as physical pain. The possibility of an accidental disclosure of a young person's mental health diagnosis and the ensuing potential for mischief and peer cruelty are real concerns. But words can also provide relief and a better understanding. Sometimes just having a name for a problem, as well as the understanding that other young people have gone through similar difficulties, can provide comfort and the beginnings of self-acceptance. We view psychiatric classification as a tool to be used in helping to deal with human problems. Like all tools, it can be used well or badly and can have good or bad effects on people's lives. We need the best tools available, and we need to use these tools well. A deficiency in either the quality of our instruments or our application of them can decrease our effectiveness.

The strengths and weaknesses of DSM-5 as a classification system in general, and the use of DSM-5 with children in particular, have received a good deal of critical attention. This circumstance is as it should be; vigorous evaluation can only benefit future attempts to portray the challenges of human adjustment more usefully. In this book, we have assumed that a decision to use DSM-5 has already been made, and we have paid little attention to the various conceptual, empirical, and practical criticisms of using DSM-5 with adults or children. Before closing, however, we want to touch at least briefly on some of the major concerns that have been advanced by various investigators and practitioners. For fuller treatment of this important area and citations of the growing literature of critical analysis of previous editions of DSM, the reader is referred to Achenbach and McConaughy (1996), Jensen and Hoagwood (1997), Scotti, Morris, McNeil, and Hawkins (1996), and Silk, Nath, Siegel, and Kendall (2000). For a critical examination of the current edition (DSM-5), see Frances (2013) and Greenberg (2013).

CONCERNS ABOUT PSYCHIATRIC CLASSIFICATION IN GENERAL

The concerns that have been expressed about the use of DSM-5 often begin with reservations about psychiatric diagnosis of children in general and then go on to the specific real or potential weaknesses of this particular system of classification. The general concerns frequently discussed include issues of inviting bias and stigmatization, unfairly portraying clients as somehow responsible for their behavior problems ("blaming the victims"), contributing to a false and premature closure of inquiry as a client is assigned a diagnosis, oversimplifying complex human problems, and ignoring important individual differences. These concerns can be voiced about any systematic classification of abnormal behavior. Potential alternative solutions include not classifying behavior at all (if it is possible), using purely idiographic or functional analyses of behavior, or identifying behavior change needs in more positive terms (idealistic or growth-based conceptualizations of behavior). DSM-5 may be used as a specific example of the problems inherent in psychiatric classification, but the concerns are often not limited to this system. It is the endeavor of classifying human problems itself that is seen as fraught with negative consequences for those we wish to assist.

In one sense these discussions are truly "academic," because we do classify people both formally and informally and will continue do so as long as there are differential assignments, treatments, learning environments, and resources to allocate. In a more fundamental sense, however, such debates are important: These concerns and exchanges serve to remind us to consider the effects of our actions. There is a link, unfortunately, between the clinical diagnosis of Intellectual Disability in a child's chart and the painful taunt of "Retard!" hurled across the playground. Although we cannot eliminate the insults by banning the diagnoses, it would be foolish to ignore the reality that our words can have many unintended consequences. Substituting new labels is only a temporary solution. A few years ago, "developmental disability" began to become the preferred phrase for children with Intellectual Disability. Within only a couple of months of reading the phrase used in this way in a professional journal, we heard on a local playground the epithet, "You DD!" It behooves us to consider our language on a regular basis and to avoid terms and phrases that have taken on prejudicial or emotionally hurtful meanings; however, real progress here requires an ongoing and honest dialogue in the society at large about behavioral differences and ways to address these challenges. DSM-5, to the degree that it is a more objective and empirically validated system of psychiatric classification than the alternatives, provides as good a foundation upon which to base this dialogue as any other.

Another significant concern is the possibility of racial or ethnic bias in psychiatric classification. Although the development of more objective diagnostic criteria almost certainly helped in this area, there was also compelling empirical evidence that problems remained in previous editions of DSM (Pavkov, Lewis, & Lyons, 1989). DSM-5 includes a Glossary of Cultural Concepts of Distress, as well as an extensive discussion of Cultural Formulation of diagnoses. The influence of these appendices on actual clinical practice remains to be seen.

Despite these efforts, many fundamental questions remain about the best ways to understand cultural differences in the classification of adjustment problems (Stein, 1993). Twenty years ago Cervantes and Arroyo (1994) discussed the use of DSM-IV with Hispanic children and adolescents and made a number of recommendations aimed at minimizing potential cultural biases in applying the classification system to this expanding segment of the population. As Cervantes and Arroyo pointed out, there were few empirical data from which to draw guidance in this area. Unfortunately, this lack of information is still the case. Novins and colleagues (1997) presented an illustration of the DSM-IV approach with Native American children. They discussed both DSM-IV's improved coverage and its continuing limitations with respect to ethnicity and cultural background. Their questions will apply equally to DSM-5. There are no absolute guidelines to apply to these challenges. Some scholars have even questioned the idea of "culture-bound syndromes" (Bartholomew, 1995). Yet few would debate the assertion that our cultural heritage affects behavior, and therefore aberrations of that behavior, in a pervasive way. Both empirical study and open dialogue are needed to promote culturally appropriate services for minorities and subgroups within the U.S. population.

CONCERNS ABOUT THE OVERALL CONCEPTUALIZATION AND STRUCTURE OF DSM-5

On a still general level, but pertaining more directly to DSM-5, are concerns about the overall conceptualization and structure of this taxonomic system. DSM-5 uses a categorical model, relies on clinical assessment, allows multiple diagnoses, and often employs polycritic criterion sets (in which, say, 6 or 9 or 3 of a list of 15 symptoms are enough to satisfy a requirement). These features have all received both positive and negative comments.

Levy, Hay, McStephen, Wood, and Waldman (1997) analyzed data from a cohort of 1,938 families and concluded that Attention-Deficit/Hyperactivity Disorder is best viewed as an extreme expression of behavior that varies along a continuum, rather than as a categorical disorder. Shaywitz, Escobar, and colleagues (1990) have raised similar concerns about "dyslexia." Questions have also been asked about depression, anxiety, substance use, social isolation, autistic thinking, reality testing, eating disturbances, sleep problems, and virtually every other difficulty formulated within DSM-5. There is some discussion of continua within DSM-5, but it remains a categorical system. For example, Autistic Spectrum Disorder is a single category that collapses several previous categories. And, even though human variability may be continuous, our responses to it are not. A child either goes to the reading resource room during third period or does not, a prescription for a stimulant medication is made or is not, counseling sessions are recommended or they are not. As long as specific dispositions are to be made, then even a continuous variable will be dichotomized in some manner: Up to a certain point, a young person continues with regular classes; if the variable is more extreme than this threshold, an alternative plan is put in motion. How best to deal with the reality that human variability may well be continuous along dimensions but our response to it will usually be of a categorical nature (e.g., go/no-go) remains a challenge.

The ultimate reliance on clinical judgment and decision making in the DSM-5 system has been commented upon several times already. It is both a strength and a weakness of DSM-5. Human judgment and decision making, guided by clear statements and objective criteria, offer the most sophisticated and subtle problem-solving solutions possible. The human mind is capable of weighing multiple factors to arrive at a conclusion; at the present time, no mechanical decision-making algorithm is presently superior to it over the range of activities covered in DSM-5. At the same time, this reliance on clinical judgment brings with it possibilities of bias, idiosyncratic decisions, errors, and intentional circumventions in the diagnostic process. Individual evaluators are responsible for the quality and accuracy of their diagnostic assignments. Ongoing education, consultation, and review of previous decisions are essential for the appropriate and accurate application of DSM-5.

Another body of misgivings about DSM-5 relates to the number of diagnostic categories and the frequent occurrence of multiple diagnoses. The system has been criticized as too complicated, with too many diagnoses between which a practitioner will not reliably make discriminations.

The usual observation that comorbidity of psychiatric diagnoses was the rule rather than the exception with DSM-IV appears to be likely to continue with DSM-5 and also causes concern. The ICD system, through most of its editions, has sought to reduce the number of behavioral classifications by an emphasis on making a single mental health diagnosis and by the use of combined categories (e.g., "mixed anxiety and depressive disorder"). The deliberate strategy of providing a wide array of behavioral classifications and of allowing concurrent diagnoses speaks to the intention of DSM-5's authors to continue to provide the most comprehensive accounting of mental health problems possible. The basic reality is that human behavior is fantastically complex and problematic manifestations are no less so, and most of us have not isolated difficulties but combinations of problems. DSM-5 attempts to mirror as fully as possible the range and nature of human behavioral problems. In doing so, it necessarily takes on a complex and elaborate form. Efforts to hold down or reduce the number of categories proceed hand in hand with efforts to achieve even finer degrees of differentiation (and hence more categories and probably more multiple categorizations).

SPECIFIC CONCERNS ABOUT DSM-5

On yet another level are specific concerns or criticisms regarding the categories, criteria, and diagnostic thresholds of DSM-5—both those carried over from DSM-IV-TR (the majority) and the new formulations being used and evaluated for the first time.

The relation between classifications of behavior problems in children versus adolescents versus adults remains a continuing concern. Many of the "child" diagnoses in DSM-IV have been absorbed into the thematic areas of diagnosis (Depressive Disorders, Anxiety Disorders, etc.) in DSM-5. Greater attention has also been given to identifying developmentally characteristic symptom manifestations within several criterion sets (e.g., Posttraumatic Stress Disorder in children and Attention-Deficit/Hyperactivity Disorder in adults). Ongoing epidemiological and general population studies continue to increase our understanding of the typical onset and course of autism, attention problems, and mood disturbances, to name only a few. Despite these efforts, the most useful boundaries and conceptualizations for capturing the difficulties of childhood and adolescence remain subjects of much contention and debate. For example, a significant amount of debate and effort again went into the multisite field trials of proposed Disruptive, Impulse-Control, and Conduct Disorder categories for DSM-5. In spite of this effort, we anticipate there will be continued dissatisfaction over the boundaries between categories (e.g., Conduct Disorder and Oppositional

Defiant Disorder) and within categories (e.g., the Predominantly Inattentive and Predominantly Hyperactive–Impulsive presentations of Attention-Deficit/Hyperactivity Disorder).

Empirical studies of a number of diagnostic categories have concluded with remarkably consistent findings: (1) Diagnostic threshold translates directly into the size of the population identified as showing a given problem; (2) a more inclusive definition increases the heterogeneity and reduces the average severity of disturbance in the population identified; and (3) in the usual absence of a "gold standard" of diagnostic correctness, there is not usually a natural break clearly demonstrating the superiority of one threshold of symptom frequency over another. As increasingly differentiated intervention and empirically supported therapy options continue to become more available, the potential costs of false-positive versus false-negative errors may play an increasing role in future reformulations of diagnostic systems. We predict that the challenge of differential diagnosis will remain an area of ongoing concern over the life of DSM-5 and that various tools and approaches to address this need will continue to appear.

The greater emphasis on clinically significant impairment incorporated into most of the diagnostic categories of DSM-5 pertaining to children and adolescents also deserves some comment. The understandable intent was to decrease false-positive diagnoses of minor or trivial problems of life as mental disorders because particular patterns of mild intensity happened to meet the "formal" diagnostic criteria. The purpose of the DSM-5 definition of Mental Disorders is clearly to identify and classify abnormal patterns of action and feelings. This emphasis requires a focus on the overall functioning of the youth. With the abandonment of DSM-IV's Axis V, the Global Assessment of Functioning (GAF) rating, there will be a need for new approaches to quantify and objectively assess adjustment and functioning in youth.

The extent of, and dependence upon, various methodologies of data collection constitute another area of continued questions regarding DSM-5. As noted earlier in this book, DSM-5 calls for formal psychological or other assessment for only a few diagnostic decisions (Intellectual Disability, Learning Disorders, Communication Disorders, certain cognitive problems). In common clinical practice, self-report instruments, behavior rating scales, and structured interviews are frequently employed in the assessment of a variety of other problem areas. Many investigators and practitioners working with youth being assessed for Attention-Deficit/Hyperactivity Disorder insist on the use of age- and gender-normed behavior ratings of core symptoms by one or more informants familiar with a child's behavior in natural life settings. Self-report and behavior rating symptom scales are being increasingly used in the evaluation of childhood and adolescent depression, anxiety, dissociative symptoms, sleep problems, conduct problems, and other areas of maladjustment and distress. Both comprehensive and domain-specific structured interviews have been developed for childhood behavior problems. All of these generally positive developments bring in their own sets of methodological issues and problems. For example, how many adult informants should complete an Attention-Deficit/Hyperactivity Disorder rating scale for a child, which scale should be used, and how should the examiner deal with discrepancies among reports? The questions are multiple, important, and often without clear and definitive answers. Auxiliary tools clearly have the potential to increase the objectivity and reliability of DSM-5 classification; realizing this potential, however, will require a great deal of empirical investigation. The availability of objective, reliable, and empirically validated diagnostic categories can only facilitate this ongoing, important work.

DID THEY GET IT RIGHT?

How should we evaluate DSM-5? This question has many possible answers. Some of the answers will become apparent only with time: Will the revised classification system be used by providers, by third-party carriers, by governmental services, by researchers, and in the lay press? DSM-5 has some serious competition out there. The National Institute of Mental Health is developing its own classification system for evaluation of research proposals seeking public funding. Some clinicians are viewing ICD-10, and eventually ICD-11, as real alternatives. It is no longer clear that DSM will be "the only game in town," as is said in the punch line to an old joke about playing in crooked card games.

As a scientific document, the question "Did they get it right?" brings up issues of reliability and validity. These issues have received significant attention since the watershed publication of DSM-III. There will no doubt be many publications presenting data on how consistently clinicians and researchers use this iteration and how well the revised categories capture essential and useful groupings of mental and behavioral challenges in children.

Although many critiques can and will be voiced about DSM-5, it is currently the best effort of a large group of highly trained, experienced, and dedicated professionals to understand how human beings get themselves into difficulty with their lives and the afflictions that life visits upon them. Countless hours were devoted to sifting through the available clinical research literature, writing and criticizing drafts, and debating strongly held positions forged from years of experience. It is useful to keep in mind that the product we hold in our hands is a group effort, which inevitably means it is a compromise. Consensus often does not mean the same thing as complete agreement. We might have wished for more transparency in the process. For some of us there might have been more to learn from the arguments and disagreements than from the final product. But the resulting document is what we have for now.

Some authors clearly believe that mental disorders will ultimately be understood in terms of neurological processes and that all emotional and behavioral disorders are based in disordered biological mechanisms. This notion is the original Kraepelinian belief. Because we do not yet have this full understanding, the phenomenological and overt descriptive categories we make use of are necessary intermediate tools. Although biological factors are clearly involved to some degree in many or most mental disorders, the extreme version of this position remains in as much doubt today as when it was formulated over a century ago. To us it appears that, at least for today, mental disorders are abstractions created by people to help make sense of the difficulties that people experience. Mental abstractions can be extremely useful, but they may or may not be "true" in any primary sense. Utility may be a better metric for evaluation than how fundamentally correct the categories are.

If DSM-5 stimulates better research into the causes and influences of behavioral adjustment, if it brings more compassionate understanding to the lives of our clients, if it allows for the development of more effective treatments of mental disorders—then it will have served well. In our opinion, the outcomes will be the ultimate answer to the question.

CONCLUDING REMARKS

It is our belief that the careful assessment of behavior and problems of behavior has contributed in a basic way to our growing understanding of adjustment and of psychopathology. As a part of this process, psychiatric classification has played and appears likely to continue to play an important role in research on behavioral and emotional problems of children and adolescents. Psychiatric classification also plays a significant procedural role in clinical activity; choices of medical, psychological, and educational interventions are increasingly being made on the basis of such classification. Although the DSM-5 system is not the only basis upon which evaluation can be conducted, and although (as this chapter has noted) it is by no means a perfect system, it is an important one. As the profession of psychology moves through the 21st century, we believe that psychologists practicing within educational settings will see an increasing application of the DSM classification system. In their recent discussion of the prevalence of childhood disorders, researchers estimate that between 20 and 25% of youth experience a significant mental health problem at some point (Ghandour, Kogan, Blumberg, Jones, & Perrin, 2012). This estimate indicates that there is a tremendous population in need of services. We think that the professional training of psychologists provides them with a good basis upon which to practice mental health classification and see this activity as a professional responsibility they will increasingly be called upon to perform. We hope this book proves to be of assistance to school psychologists and other child clinical professionals who are beginning to function in this additional role.

References

Abikoff, H., & Klein, R. G. (1992). Attention-deficit hyperactivity and conduct disorder: Comorbidity and implications for treatment. *Journal of Consulting and Clinical Psychology, 60*, 881–892.

Achenbach, T. M., & McConaughy, S. H. (1996). Relations between DSM-IV and empirically based assessment. *School Psychology Review, 25*, 329–341.

Adams, G. B., Waas, G. A., March, J. S., & Smith, M. C. (1994). Obsessive–compulsive disorder in children and adolescents: The role of the school psychologist in identification, assessment, and treatment. *School Psychology Quarterly, 9*, 274–294.

Aman, M. G., Hammer, D., & Rojahn, J. (1993). Mental retardation. In T. H. Ollendick & M. Hersen (Eds.), *Handbook of child and adolescent assessment* (pp. 321–345). Needham Heights, MA: Allyn & Bacon.

Aman, M. G., Pejeau, C., Osborne, P., Rojahn, J., & Handen, B. (1996). Four-year follow-up of children with low intelligence and ADHD. *Research in Developmental Disabilities, 17*, 417–432.

American Academy of Sleep Medicine. (2014). *International classification of sleep disorders: Diagnostic and coding manual* (3rd ed.). Darien, IL: American Academy of Sleep Medicine.

American Psychiatric Association. (1968). *Diagnostic and statistical manual of mental disorders* (2nd ed.). Washington, DC: Author.

American Psychiatric Association. (1980). *Diagnostic and statistical manual of mental disorders* (3rd ed.). Washington, DC: Author.

American Psychiatric Association. (1987). *Diagnostic and statistical manual of mental disorders* (3rd ed., rev.). Washington, DC: Author.

American Psychiatric Association. (1994). *Diagnostic and statistical manual of mental disorders* (4th ed.). Washington, DC: Author.
American Psychiatric Association. (2000). *Diagnostic and statistical manual of mental disorders* (4th ed., text rev.). Washington, DC: Author.
American Psychiatric Association. (2013a). *Desk reference to the diagnostic criteria from DSM-5*. Arlington, VA: Author.
American Psychiatric Association. (2013b). *Diagnostic and statistical manual of mental disorders* (5th ed.). Arlington, VA: Author.
American Psychological Association. (2007). Record keeping guidelines. *American Psychologist, 62*, 993–1004.
American Sleep Disorders Association. (1997). *The international classification of sleep disorders, revised.* Rochester, MN: Author.
American Speech–Language–Hearing Association. (2012). ASHA's recommended revisions to DSM-5: June 2012 comments. Retrieved March 16, 2015, from *www.asha.org.*
Ani, C., Reading, R., Lynn, R., Forlee, S., & Garralda, E. (2013). Incidence and 12-month outcome of non-transient childhood conversion disorder in the UK and Ireland. *British Journal of Psychiatry, 202,* 413–418.
Applegate, B., Lahey, B. B., Hart, E. L., Biederman, J., Hynd, G. W., Barkley, R. A., et al. (1997). Validity of the age-of-onset criterion for ADHD: A report from the DSM-IV field trials. *Journal of the American Academy of Child and Adolescent Psychiatry, 36*, 1211–1221.
Armstrong, J. G., Putnam, F. W., Carlson, E. B., Libero, D. Z., & Smith, S. R. (1997). Development and validation of a measure of adolescent dissociation: The Adolescent Dissociative Experiences Scale. *Journal of Nervous and Mental Disease, 185*, 491–497.
Asarnow, J. R. (1994). Annotation: Childhood-onset schizophrenia. *Journal of Child Psychiatry and Psychology, 35*, 1345–1371.
Asarnow, R. F. (2013). Childhood schizophrenia. In T. P. Beauchaine & S. P. Hinshaw (Eds.), *Child and adolescent psychopathology* (4th ed., pp. 685–713). Hoboken, NJ: Wiley.
Atkins, M. S., McKay, M. M., Talbott, E., & Arvanitis, P. (1996). DSM-IV diagnosis of conduct disorder and oppositional defiant disorder: Implications and guidelines for school mental health teams. *School Psychology Review, 25*, 274–283.
August, G. J., & Garfinkel, B. D. (1989). Behavioral and cognitive subtypes of ADHD. *Journal of the American Academy of Child and Adolescent Psychiatry, 28*, 739–748.
Babor, T. F., & Caetano, R. (2006). Subtypes of substance dependence and abuse: Implications for diagnostic classification and empirical research. *Addiction, 101,* 104–110.
Barkley, R. A. (1990). *Attention-deficit hyperactivity disorder: A handbook for diagnosis and treatment.* New York: Guilford Press.
Barkley, R. A. (1991). Diagnosis and assessment of attention-deficit hyperactivity disorder. *Comprehensive Mental Health Care, 1*, 27–43.

Barkley, R. A. (2015). Psychological assessment of children with ADHD. In R. A. Barkley (Ed.), *Attention-deficit/hyperactivity disorder: A handbook for diagnosis and treatment* (4th ed., pp. 455–474). New York: Guilford Press.

Barkley, R. A., & Biederman, J. (1997). Toward a broader definition of the age-of-onset criterion for attention-deficit/hyperactivity disorder. *Journal of the American Academy of Child and Adolescent Psychiatry, 36*, 1204–1210.

Bartholomew, R. E. (1995). Culture-bound syndromes as fakery. *Skeptical Inquirer, 19*, 36–41.

Bauermeister, J. J., Canino, G., Polanczyk, G., & Rohde, L. A. (2010). ADHD across cultures: Is there evidence for a bidimensional organization of symptoms? *Journal of Clinical Child and Adolescent Psychology, 39*, 362–372.

Baumgaertel, A., Wolraich, M. L., & Dietrich, M. (1995). Comparison of diagnostic criteria for attention-deficit disorders in a German elementary school sample. *Journal of the American Academy of Child and Adolescent Psychiatry, 34*, 629–638.

Beck, A. T., Freeman, A., & Associates. (1990). *Cognitive therapy of personality disorders*. New York: Guilford Press.

Begali, V. (1992). *Head injury in children and adolescents: A resource and review for school and allied professionals*. Brandon, VT: Clinical Psychology.

Bernstein, D. P., Cohen, P., Velez, C. N., Schwab-Stone, M., Siever, L. J., & Shinsato, L. (1993). Prevalence and stability of the DSM-III-R personality disorders in a community-based survey of adolescents. *American Journal of Psychiatry, 150*, 1237–1243.

Bernstein, G. A., & Borchardt, C. M. (1991). Anxiety disorders of childhood and adolescence: A critical review. *Journal of the American Academy of Child and Adolescent Psychiatry, 30*, 519–532.

Biederman, J. (1991). Attention-deficit hyperactivity disorder (ADHD). *Annals of Clinical Psychiatry, 3*, 9–22.

Biederman, J. (1997). Is there a childhood form of bipolar disorder? *Harvard Mental Health Letter, 13*, 8.

Biederman, J., Faraone, S. V., Marrs, A., Moore, P., Garcia, J., Ablon, S., et al. (1997). Panic disorder and agoraphobia in consecutively referred children and adolescents. *Journal of the American Academy of Child and Adolescent Psychiatry, 36*, 214–223.

Biederman, J., Faraone, S. V., Milberger, S., Jetton, J. G., Chen, L., Mick, E., et al. (1996). Is childhood oppositional defiant disorder a precursor to adolescent conduct disorder?: Findings from a four-year follow-up study of children with ADHD. *Journal of the American Academy of Child and Adolescent Psychiatry, 35*, 1193–1204.

Birmaher, B., Gill, M. K., Axelson, D. A., Goldstein, B. I., Goldstein, T. R., Yu, H., et al. (2014). Longitudinal trajectories and associated baseline predictors in youths with bipolar spectrum disorders. *American Journal of Psychiatry, 171,* 990–999.

Birmaher, B., Khetarpal, S., Brent, D., Cully, M., Balach, L., Kaufman, J., et al. (1997). The Screen for Child Anxiety Related Emotional Disorders (SCARED): Scale construction and psychometric characteristics. *Journal of the American Academy of Child and Adolescent Psychiatry, 36,* 545–553.

Birmaher, B., Ryan, N. D., Williamson, D. E., Brent, D. A., Kaufman, J., Dahl, R. E., et al. (1996). Childhood and adolescent depression: A review of the past 10 years: Part I. *Journal of the American Academy of Child and Adolescent Psychiatry, 35,* 1427–1439.

Bleiberg, E. (1994). Borderline disorders in children and adolescents: The concept, the diagnosis, and the controversies. *Bulletin of the Menninger Clinic, 58,* 169–196.

Bloch, M. H., Panza, K. E., Grant, J. E., Pittenger, C., & Leckman, J. F. (2013). N-acetylcysteine in the treatment of pediatric trichotillomania: A randomized, double-blind, placebo-controlled add-on trial. *Journal of the American Academy of Child and Adolescent Psychiatry, 52,* 231–240.

Blom, M., & Oberink, R. (2012). The validity of the DSM-IV PTSD criteria in children and adolescents: A review. *Clinical Child Psychology and Psychiatry, 17,* 571–601.

Boyson, G. A. (2011). The scientific status of childhood dissociative identity disorder: A review of published research. *Psychotherapy and Psychosomatics, 80,* 329–334.

Bradley, S. J., & Zucker, K. J. (1997). Gender identity disorder: A review of the past 10 years. *Journal of the American Academy of Child and Adolescent Psychiatry, 36,* 872–880.

Bray, M. A., Kehle, T. J., & Theodore, L. A. (2014). Best practices in the assessment and remediation of communication disorders. In P. L. Harrison & A. Thomas (Eds.), *Best practices in school psychology: Data-based and collaborative decision making* (pp. 355–365). Bethesda, MD: National Association of School Psychologists.

Bregman, J. D. (1991). Current developments in the understanding of mental retardation: Part II. *Psychopathology, 30,* 861–872.

Brown, G., Chadwick, O., Shaffer, D., Rutter, M., & Traub, M. (1981). A prospective study of children with head injuries: III. Psychiatric sequelae. *Psychological Medicine, 11,* 63–78.

Bryant-Waugh, R., & Lask, B. (1995). Annotation: Eating disorders in children. *Journal of Child Psychiatry and Psychology, 36,* 191–202.

Burke, J. D., Boylan, K., Rowe, R., Duku, E., Stepp, S. D., Hipwell, A. E., et al. (2014). Identifying the irritability dimension of ODD: Application of a modified bifactor model across five large community samples of children. *Journal of Abnormal Psychology, 123,* 841–851.

Burns, G. L., Walsh, J. A., Owens, S. M., & Snell, J. (1997). Internal validity of attention-deficit/hyperactivity disorder, oppositional defiant disorder, and overt conduct disorder symptoms in young children: Implications from teacher ratings for a dimensional approach to symptom validity. *Journal of Clinical Child Psychology, 26*, 266–275.

Caetano, R., & Babor, T. F. (2006). Diagnosis of alcohol dependence in epidemiological surveys: An epidemic of youthful alcohol dependence or a case of measurement error? *Addiction, 101*, 111–114.

Cahill, L. M., Murdoch, B. E., & Theodoros, D. G. (2005). Articulatory function following traumatic brain injury in childhood: A perceptual and instrumental analysis. *Brain Injury, 19*(1), 55–79.

Campbell, M., & Malone, R. P. (1991). Mental retardation and psychiatric disorders. *Hospital and Community Psychiatry, 42*, 374–379.

Cantwell, D., & Baker, L. (1987). *Developmental speech and language disorders*. New York: Guilford Press.

Cantwell, D., Lewinsohn, P. M., Rohde, P., & Seeley, J. R. (1997). Correspondence between adolescent report and parent report of psychiatric diagnostic date. *Journal of the American Academy of Child and Adolescent Psychiatry, 36*, 610–619.

Carbone, D., Schmidt, L. A., Cunningham, C. C., McHolm, A. E., Edison, S., St. Pierre, J., et al. (2010). Behavioral and socio-emotional functioning in children with selective mutism: A comparison with anxious and typically developing children across multiple informants. *Journal of Abnormal Child Psychology, 38*, 1057–1067.

Carlson, G. A., & Meyer, S. E. (2006). Phenomenology and diagnosis of bipolar disorder in children, adolescents, and adults: Complexities and developmental issues. *Development and Psychopathology, 18*, 939–969.

Carney, J., & Schoenbrodt, L. (1994). Educational implications of traumatic brain injury. *Pediatric Annals, 23*, 47–52.

Carpenter, W. T., Heinrichs, D. W., & Wagman, A. M. I. (1988). Deficit and nondeficit forms of schizophrenia: The concept. *American Journal of Psychiatry, 145*, 578–583.

Carr, A. (2009). Bipolar disorder in young people: Description, assessment, and evidence-based treatment. *Developmental Neurorehabilitation, 12*, 427–441.

Çelik, F. H., Aktepe, E., & Kocaman, O. (2014). Pathological fire setting behavior in children and adolescents. *TAF Preventive Medicine Bulletin, 13*, 245–256.

Cervantes, R. C., & Arroyo, W. (1994). DSM-IV: Implications for Hispanic children and adolescents. *Hispanic Journal of Behavioral Sciences, 16*, 8–27.

Christian, R. E., Frick, P. J., Hill, N. L., Tyler, L., & Frazer, D. R. (1997). Psychopathy and conduct problems in children: II. Implications for subtyping children with conduct problems. *Journal of the American Academy of Child and Adolescent Psychiatry, 36*, 233–241.

Cicchetti, D., & Toth, S. L. (1998). The development of depression in children and adolescents. *American Psychologist, 53*, 221–241.

Clarizio, H. R., & Payette, K. (1990). A survey of school psychologists' perspectives and practices with childhood depression. *Psychology in the Schools, 27*, 57–63.

Cline, D. H. (1990). A legal analysis of policy initiatives to exclude handicapped/disruptive students from special education. *Behavioral Disorders, 15*, 159–173.

Cohen, N. J. (2001). *Language impairment and psychopathology in infants, children, and adolescents.* Thousand Oaks, CA: Sage.

Cohen-Kettenis, P. T., & van Goozen, S. H. M. (1997). Sex reassignment of adolescent transsexuals: A follow-up study. *Journal of the American Academy of Child and Adolescent Psychiatry, 36*, 263–271.

Colker, R., Shaywitz, S., Shaywitz, B., & Simon, J. (2014). Comments on proposed DSM-5 criteria for specific learning disorder from a legal and medical/scientific perspective. Retrieved from *http://dyslexia.yale.edu/CommentsDSM5ColkerShaywitzSimon.pdf.*

Council for Children with Behavioral Disorders. (1987). Position paper on definition and identification of students with behavioral disorders. *Behavioral Disorders, 13*, 9–19.

Creak, E. M. (1961). Schizophrenic syndrome in children: Progress of a working party. *Cerebral Palsy Bulletin, 3*, 501–503.

Creak, E. M. (1963). Childhood psychosis. *British Journal of Psychiatry, 109*, 84–89.

Crowley, T. J. (2006). Adolescents and substance-related disorders: Research agenda to guide decisions on *Diagnostic and Statistical Manual of Mental Disorders*, fifth edition (DSM-V). *Addiction, 101*, 115–124.

Cummings, C. M., Caporino, N. E., & Kendall, P. C. (2014). Comorbidity of anxiety and depression in children and adolescents: 20 years after. *Psychological Bulletin, 140*, 816–845.

Davies, S. C. (2014). Best practices in working with children with traumatic brain injuries. In P. L. Harrison & A. Thomas (Eds.), *Best practices in school psychology: Systems-level services* (pp. 405–421). Bethesda, MD: National Association of School Psychologists.

Davila, R. R., Williams, M. L., & MacDonald, J. T. (1991, September 16). *Clarification of policy to address the needs of children with attention-deficit disorders within general and/or special education* [Memorandum]. Washington, DC: U.S. Department of Education, Office of Special Education and Rehabilitative Services.

Deykin, E. Y., & Buka, S. L. (1997). Prevalence and risk factors for posttraumatic stress disorder among chemically dependent adolescents. *American Journal of Psychiatry, 154*, 752–757.

Doll, B. (1996). Prevalence of psychiatric disorders in children and youth: An agenda for advocacy by school psychology. *School Psychology Quarterly, 11*, 20–47.

Dummit, E. S., III, Klein, R. G., Tancer, N. K., Asche, B., Martin, J., & Fairbanks, J. A. (1997). Systematic assessment of 50 children with selective mutism. *Journal of the American Academy of Child and Adolescent Psychiatry, 36*, 653–660.

DuPaul, G. J., Stoner, G., & O'Reilly, M. J. (2014). Best practices in classroom interventions for attention problems. In P. L. Harrison & A. Thomas (Eds.), *Best practices in school psychology: Student-level services* (pp. 335–347). Bethesda, MD: National Association of School Psychologists.

Einfeld, S. L., & Aman, M. (1995). Issues in the taxonomy of psychopathology in mental retardation. *Journal of Autism and Developmental Disorders, 25*, 143–167.

Einfeld, S. L., Ellis, L. A., & Emerson, E. (2011). Comorbidity of intellectual disability and mental disorder in children and adolescents: A systematic review. *Journal of Intellectual and Developmental Disability, 36*, 137–143.

Elliott, C., Pruett, S., Vaal, J., Agner, J., Havey, M., Boyd, L., et al. (1993). *Best practices for third party reimbursement.* Bloomingdale: Illinois School Psychologists Association.

Emslie, G. J., Kennard, B. D., & Kowatch, R. A. (1995). Affective disorders in children: Diagnosis and management. *Journal of Child Neurology, 10*(Suppl. 1), S42–S49.

Erk, R. R. (1995). The evolution of attention-deficit disorders terminology. *Elementary School Guidance and Counseling, 29*, 243–248.

Ewing-Cobbs, L., Miner, M. E., Fletcher, J. M., & Levin, H. S. (1989). Intellectual, motor, and language sequelae following closed head injury in infants and preschoolers. *Journal of Pediatric Psychology, 14*, 531–547.

Faraone, S. V., Biederman, J., Mennin, D., Wozniak, J., & Spencer, T. (1997). Attention-deficit/hyperactivity disorder with bipolar disorder: A familial subtype? *Journal of the American Academy of Child and Adolescent Psychiatry, 36*, 1378–1387.

Faul, M., Xu, L., Wald, M. M., & Coronado, V. G. (2010). *Traumatic brain injury in the United States: Emergency department visits, hospitalizations and deaths 2002–2006.* Atlanta, GA: Centers for Disease Control and Prevention, National Center for Injury Prevention and Control.

Fauman, M. A. (1994). *Study guide to DSM-IV.* Washington, DC: American Psychiatric Press.

Fay, G. C., Jaffe, K. M., Polissar, N. L., Liao, S., Rivara, J. B., & Martin, K. M. (1994). Outcome of pediatric traumatic brain injury at three years: A cohort study. *Archives of Physical Medicine and Rehabilitation, 75*, 733–741.

First, M. B. (2014). *DSM-5 handbook of differential diagnosis* [Electronic resource]. Arlington, VA: American Psychiatric Publishing.

Fitzgerald, M. M., & Cohen, J. A. (2012). Trauma-focused cognitive behavior therapy for school psychologists. *Journal of Applied School Psychology, 28*, 294–315.

Flanagan, D. P., & Alfonso, V. C. (2010). *Essentials of specific learning disability identification.* Hoboken, NJ: Wiley.

Flessner, C. A. (2011). Cognitive-behavioral therapy for childhood repetitive behavior disorders: Tic disorders and trichotillomania. *Child and Adolescent Psychiatric Clinics of North America, 20*, 319–328.

Fletcher, J. M., Ewing-Cobbs, L., Miner, M. E., Levin, H. S., & Eisenberg, H. M. (1990). Behavioral changes after closed head injury in children. *Journal of Consulting and Clinical Psychology, 58*, 93–98.

Fletcher-Flinn, C., Elmes, H., & Strugnell, D. (1997). Visual–perceptual and phonological factors in the acquisition of literacy among children with congenital developmental coordination disorder. *Developmental Medicine and Child Neurology, 39*, 158–166.

Forness, S. R., & Knitzer, J. (1990). A new proposed definition and terminology to replace "serious emotional disturbance" in Individuals with Disabilities Education Act. *School Psychology Review, 21*, 12–20.

Frances, A. (2010). Increasing the age at onset for ADHD? *American Journal of Psychiatry, 167*, 718.

Frances, A. (2013). *Saving normal: An insider's revolt against out-of-control psychiatric diagnosis, DSM-5, big pharma, and the medicalization of ordinary life*. New York: Morrow.

Francis, G., Last, C. G., & Strauss, C. C. (1987). Expression of separation anxiety disorder: The roles of age and gender. *Child Psychiatry and Human Development, 18*, 82–89.

Francis, G., Last, C. G., & Strauss, C. C. (1992). Avoidant disorder and social phobia in children and adolescents. *Journal of the American Academy of Child and Adolescent Psychiatry, 31*, 1086–1089.

Frick, P. J., Barry, C.T., & Kamphaus, R. W. (2009). *Clinical assessment of child and adolescent personality and behavior* (3rd ed.) New York: Springer.

Frick, P. J., Kamphaus, R. W., Lahey, B. B., Loeber, R., Christ, M. A. G., Hart, E. L., et al. (1991). Academic underachievement and the disruptive behavior disorders. *Journal of Consulting and Clinical Psychology, 59*, 289–294.

Frick, P. J., Lahey, B. B., Applegate, B., Kerdyck, L., Ollendick, T., Hynd, G. W., et al. (1994). DSM-IV field trials for the disruptive behavior disorders: Symptom utility estimates. *Journal of the American Academy of Child and Adolescent Psychiatry, 33*, 529–539.

Fritz, G., Fritsch, S., & Hagino, O. (1997). Somatoform disorders in children and adolescents: A review of the past 10 years. *Journal of the American Academy of Child and Adolescent Psychiatry, 36*, 1329–1339.

Garber, J., & Weersing, V. R. (2010). Comorbidity of anxiety and depression in youth: Implications for treatment and prevention. *Clinical Psychology: Science and Practice, 17*, 293–306.

Gaub, M., & Carlson, C. L. (1997). Behavioral characteristics of DSM-IV ADHD subtypes in a school-based population. *Journal of Abnormal Child Psychology, 25*, 103–111.

Geller, B., & Luby, J. (1997). Child and adolescent bipolar disorder: A review of the past 10 years. *Journal of the American Academy of Child and Adolescent Psychiatry, 36*, 1168–1176.

Geller, B., Sun, K., Zimerman, B., Luby, J., Frazier, J., & Williams, M. (1995). Complex and rapid-cycling in bipolar children and adolescents: A preliminary study. *Journal of Affective Disorders, 34*, 259–268.

Ghandour, R. M., Kogan, M. D., Blumberg, S. J., Jones, J. R., & Perrin, J. M. (2012). Mental health conditions among school-aged children: Geographic and sociodemographic patterns in prevalence and treatment. *Journal of Developmental and Behavioral Pediatrics, 33*, 42–54.

Giaconia, R. M., Reinherz, H. Z., Silverman, A. B., Pakiz, B., Frost, A. K., & Cohen, E. (1995). Traumas and posttraumatic stress disorder in a community population of older adolescents. *Journal of the American Academy of Child and Adolescent Psychiatry, 34*, 1369–1380.

Giedd, J. N., Swedo, S. S., Lowe, C. H., & Rosenthal, N. E. (1998). Case series: Pediatric seasonal affective disorder: A follow-up report. *Journal of the American Academy of Child and Adolescent Psychiatry, 37*, 218–220.

Glaros, A. G., & Melamed, B. G. (1992). Bruxism in children: Etiology and treatment. *Applied and Preventive Psychology, 1*, 191–199.

Goldman, S. J., D'Angelo, E. J., Demaso, D. R., & Mezzacappa, E. (1992). Physical and sexual abuse histories among children with borderline personality disorder. *American Journal of Psychiatry, 149*, 1723–1726.

Goodheart, C. D. (2014). *A primer for ICD-10-CM users.* Washington, DC: American Psychological Association.

Greenberg, G. (2013). *The book of woe: The DSM and the unmaking of psychiatry.* New York: Blue Rider Press.

Gresham, F. M., MacMillan, D. L., & Bocian, K. M. (1998). Agreement between school study team decisions and authoritative definitions in classifications of students at-risk for mild disabilities. *School Psychology Quarterly, 13*, 181–191.

Gresham, F. M., MacMillan, D. L., & Siperstein, G. N. (1995). Critical analysis of the 1992 AAMR definition: Implications for school psychology. *School Psychology Quarterly, 10*, 1–19.

Grilo, C. M., Walker, M. L., Becker, D. E., Edell, W. S., & McGlashan, T. H. (1997). Personality disorders in adolescents with major depression, substance use disorders, and coexisting major depression and substance use disorders. *Journal of Consulting and Clinical Psychology, 65*, 328–332.

Grossman, H. (1983). *Classification in mental retardation* (3rd rev.). Washington, DC: American Association on Mental Deficiency.

Gullone, E. (2000). The development of normal fear: A century of research. *Clinical Psychology Review, 20*, 429–451.

Guzder, J., Paris, J., Zelkowitz, P., & Marchessault, K. (1996). Risk factors for borderline pathology in children. *Journal of the American Academy of Child and Adolescent Psychiatry, 35*, 26–33.

Hall, A., Slim, E., Hawker, F., & Salmond, C. (1984). Anorexia nervosa:

Long-term outcome in 50 female patients. *British Journal of Psychiatry, 145*, 407–413.

Halperin, J. M., Matier, K., Bedi, G., Sharma, V., & Newcorn, J. H. (1992). Specificity of inattention, impulsivity, and hyperactivity to the diagnosis of attention-deficit/hyperactivity disorder. *Journal of the American Academy of Child and Adolescent Psychiatry, 31*, 190–196.

Halperin, J. M., Newcorn, J. H., Sharma, V., Healey, J. M., Wolf, L. E., Pascualvaca, D. M., et al. (1990). Inattentive and noninattentive ADHD children: Do they constitute a unitary group? *Journal of Abnormal Child Psychology, 18*, 437–449.

Hardman, M. L., Drew, C. J., & Egan, M. W. (2014). *Human exceptionality: School, community, and family* (11th ed.). Belmont, CA: Wadsworth Cengage Learning.

Harris, J. C. (2006). *Intellectual disability: Understanding its development, causes, classification, evaluation, and treatment*. New York: Oxford University Press.

Hart, C., & Ksir, C. (2012). *Drugs, society, and human behavior* (15th ed.). New York: McGraw-Hill.

Hayward, C., Killen, J. D., Kramer, H. C., Blair-Greiner, A., Strachowski, D., Cunning, D., et al. (1997). Assessment and phenomenology of nonclinical panic attacks in adolescent girls. *Journal of Anxiety Disorders, 11*, 17–32.

Heber, R. (1959). A manual on terminology and classification in mental retardation. *American Journal of Mental Deficiency, 56*(Suppl. 64), 1–111.

Heber, R. (1961). Modifications in the manual on terminology and classification in mental retardation. *American Journal of Mental Deficiency, 65*, 499–500.

Hellgren, L., Gillberg, I. C., Bahenholm, A., & Gillberg, C. (1994). Children with deficits in attention, motor control and perception (DAMP) almost grown up: Psychiatric and personality disorders at age 16 years. *Journal of Child Psychiatry and Psychology, 35*, 1255–1271.

Henderson, S. E., Barnett, A., & Henderson, L. (1994). Visuospatial difficulties and clumsiness: On the interpretation of conjoined deficits. *Journal of Child Psychiatry and Psychology, 35*, 961–969.

Herbert, J. (1995). An overview of the current status of social phobia. *Applied and Preventive Psychology, 4*, 39–51.

Hess, R. S., Pejic, V., & Castejon, K. S. (2014). Best practices in delivering culturally responsive, tiered-level supports for youth with behavioral challenges. In P. L. Harrison & A. Thomas (Eds.), *Best practices in school psychology: Student-level services* (pp. 321–334). Bethesda, MD: National Association of School Psychologists.

Hinshaw, S. P. (1992). Academic underachievement, attention deficits, and aggression: Comorbidity and implications for intervention. *Journal of Consulting and Clinical Psychology, 60*, 893–903.

Horowitz, M., Siegel, B., Holen, A., Bonanno, G. A., Milbrath, C., & Stinson,

C. H. (1997). Diagnostic criteria for complicated grief disorder. *American Journal of Psychiatry, 154*, 904–910.

Individuals with Disabilities Education Improvement Act of 2004. Public Law No. 108-446, 20 U. S. C. §§ 1400 et seq. (2004). Amendments to Individuals with Disabilities Education Act of 1990. Public Law No. 101-476, 20 U. S. C. § 1401 et seq.

Isaac, G. (1991). Bipolar disorder in prepubertal children in a special education setting: Is it rare? *Journal of Clinical Psychiatry, 52*, 165–168.

Jacobson, J. W. (1982). Problem behavior and psychiatric impairment in a developmentally disabled population: I. Behavior frequency. *Applied Research in Mental Retardation, 3*, 121–139.

Jensen, P. S., & Hoagwood, K. (1997). The book of names: DSM-IV in context. *Development and Psychopathology, 9*, 231–249.

Jordan, F. M., Murdoch, B. E., Buttsworth, D. L., & Hudson-Tennent, L. J. (1995). Speech and language performance of brain-injured children. *Aphasiology, 9*, 23–32.

Jordan, F. M., Ozanne, A. E., & Murdoch, B. E. (1988). Long-term speech and language disorders subsequent to closed head injury in children. *Brain Injury, 2*, 179–185.

Jordan, F. M., Ozanne, A. E., & Murdoch, B. E. (1990). Performance of closed head-injured children on a naming task. *Brain Injury, 4*, 27–32.

Kashani, J. H., Allan, W. D., Beck, N. C., Jr., Bledsoe, Y., & Reid, J. C. (1997). Dysthymic disorder in clinically referred preschool children. *Journal of the American Academy of Child and Adolescent Psychiatry, 36*, 1426–1433.

Kashani, J. H., Holcomb, W. R., & Orvaschel, H. (1986). Depression and depressive symptoms in preschool children from the general population. *American Journal of Psychiatry, 143*, 1138–1143.

Katon, W. (1993). Somatization disorder, hypochondriasis, and conversion disorder. In D. Dunner (Ed.), *Current psychiatric therapy* (pp. 314–320). Philadelphia: Saunders.

Kay, S. R. (1989). Cognitive battery for differential diagnosis of mental retardation vs. psychosis. *Research in Developmental Disabilities, 10*, 251–260.

Kearney, C., Albano, A. M., Eisen, A. R., Allan, W. D., & Barlow, D. H. (1997). The phenomenology of panic disorder in youngsters: An empirical study of a clinical sample. *Journal of Anxiety Disorders, 11*, 49–62.

Keeton, C. P., & Budinger, M. C. (2012). Social phobia and selective mutism. *Child and Adolescent Psychiatric Clinics, 21*, 621–641.

Keller, M. B. (1994). Course, outcome and impact on the community. *Acta Psychiatrica Scandinavica, 89*, 24–34.

Kessler, R. C., Avenevoli, S., Costello, J., Georgiades, K., Green, J. G., Gruber, M. J., et al. (2012). Prevalence, persistence, and sociodemographic correlates of DSM-IV disorders in the National Comorbidity Survey Replication Adolescent Supplement. *Archives of General Psychiatry, 69*, 372–380.

Kessler, R. C., Berglund, P., Demler, O., Jin, R., Merikangas, K. R., & Walters, E. E. (2005). Lifetime prevalence and age-of-onset distributions of DSM-IV disorders in the National Comorbidity Survey Replication. *Archives of General Psychiatry, 62,* 593–602.

Khan, A., Cowan, C., & Roy, A. (1997). Personality disorders in people with learning disabilities: A community survey. *Journal of Intellectual Disability Research, 41,* 324–330.

King, B. H., DeAntonio, C., McCracken, J. T., Forness, S. R., & Ackerland, V. (1994). Psychiatric consultation in severe and profound mental retardation. *American Journal of Psychiatry, 151,* 1802–1808.

King, B. H., State, M. W., Shah, B., Davanzo, P., & Dykens, E. (1997). Mental retardation: A review of the past 10 years: Part 1. *Journal of the American Academy of Child and Adolescent Psychiatry, 36,* 1656–1663.

King, S., Waschbusch, D. A., Pelham, W. E., Jr., Frankland, B. W., Andrade, B. F., Jacques, S., et al. (2009). Social information processing in elementary-school-aged children with ADHD: Mediator effects and comparisons with typical children. *Journal of Abnormal Child Psychology, 37,* 579–589.

Kirk, S. A., & Kutchins, H. (1992). *The selling of DSM: The rhetoric of science in psychiatry.* New York: Aldine de Gruyter.

Knight, J. R., Sherritt, L., Shrier, L. A., Harris, S. K., & Chang, G. (2002). Validity of the CRAFFT substance abuse screening test among adolescent clinic patients. *Archives of Pediatric Adolescent Medicine, 156,* 607–614.

Knights, R. M., Ivan, L. P., Ventureyra, E. C. G., Bentivoglio, C., Stoddart, C., Winogron, W., et al. (1991). The effects of head injury in children on neuropsychological and behavioral functioning. *Brain Injury, 5,* 339–351.

Koerner, K., Kohlenberg, R. J., & Parker, C. R. (1996). Diagnosis of personality disorder: A radical behavioral alternative. *Journal of Consulting and Clinical Psychology, 64,* 1169–1176.

Kopp, S., & Gillberg, C. (1997). Selective mutism: A population-based study: A research note. *Journal of Child Psychology and Psychiatry, 38,* 257–262.

Kronenberger, W. G., & Meyer, R. G. (2001). *The child clinician's handbook* (2nd ed.). Boston: Allyn & Bacon.

Kutchins, H., & Kirk, S. A. (1995). DSM-IV: Does bigger and newer mean better? *Harvard Mental Health Letter, 11,* 4–6.

Lahey, B. B., Applegate, B., McBurnett, K., Biederman, J., Greenhill, L., Hynd, G. W., et al. (1994). DSM-IV field trials for attention-deficit/hyperactivity disorder in children and adolescents. *American Journal of Psychiatry, 151,* 1673–1685.

Lahey, B. B., Loeber, R., Quay, H. C., Frick, P. J., & Grimm, J. (1992). Oppositional–defiant and conduct disorders: Issues to be resolved in DSM-IV. *Journal of the American Academy of Child and Adolescent Psychiatry, 31,* 539–545.

Lahey, B. B., Schaughency, E., Hynd, G., Carlson, C., & Nieves, N. (1987).

Attention-deficit disorder with and without hyperactivity: Comparison of behavioral characteristics of clinic-referred children. *Journal of the American Academy of Child Psychiatry, 26*, 718–723.

Last, C. G., Francis, G., Hersen, M., Kazdin, A. E., & Strauss, C. C. (1987). Separation anxiety and school phobia: A comparison using DSM-III criteria. *American Journal of Psychiatry, 144*, 653–657.

Lehmkuhl, G., Blanz, B., Lehmkuhl, U., & Braum-Scharm, H. (1989). Conversion disorder (DSM-III 300.11): Symptomatology and course in childhood and adolescence. *European Archives of Psychiatry and Neurological Sciences, 238*, 155–160.

Leibenluft, E., Cohen, P., Gorrindo, T., Brook, J. S., & Pine, D. S. (2006). Chronic versus episodic irritability in youth: A community-based, longitudinal study of clinical and diagnostic associations. *Journal of Child and Adolescent Psychopharmacology, 16*, 456–466.

Levy, E., Hay, D. A., McStephen, M., Wood, C., & Waldman, I. (1997). Attention-deficit/hyperactivity disorder: A category or a continuum? Genetic analysis of a large-scale twin study. *Journal of the American Academy of Child and Adolescent Psychiatry, 36*, 737–744.

Lewinsohn, P. M., Rohde, P., Seeley, J. R., & Klein, D. N. (1997). Axis II psychopathology as a function of Axis I disorders in childhood and adolescence. *Journal of the American Academy of Child and Adolescent Psychiatry, 36*, 1752–1759.

Lewis, D. O., Lewis, M., Unger, L., & Goldman, C. (1984). Conduct disorder and its synonyms: Diagnoses of dubious validity and usefulness. *American Journal of Psychiatry, 141*, 514–519.

Lewis, M. (1996). Borderline features in childhood disorders. In F. R. Volkmar (Ed.), *Psychoses and pervasive developmental disorders in childhood and adolescence* (pp. 103–123). Washington, DC: American Psychiatric Press.

Linehan, M. M. (1993). *Cognitive-behavioral treatment of borderline personality disorder.* New York: Guilford Press.

Loeber, R., Lahey, B. B., & Thomas, C. (1991). Diagnostic conundrum of oppositional–defiant disorder and conduct disorder. *Journal of Abnormal Psychology, 100*, 379–390.

Lovaas, I., Newsom, C., & Hickman, C. (1987). Self-stimulatory behavior and perceptual reinforcement. *Journal of Applied Behavior Analysis, 20*, 45–68.

Ludolph, P. S., Westen, D., Misle, B., Jackson, A., Wixom, J., & Wiss, F. C. (1990). The borderline diagnosis in adolescents: Symptoms and developmental history. *American Journal of Psychiatry, 147*, 470–476.

Lynam, D. R. (1996). Early identification of the chronic offender: Who is the fledgling psychopath? *Psychological Bulletin, 120*, 209–234.

Lynskey, M., & Fergusson, D. M. (1995). Childhood conduct problems, attention-deficit behaviors, and adolescent alcohol, tobacco, and illicit drug use. *Journal of Abnormal Child Psychology, 23*, 281–302.

MacMillan, D. L., Gresham, F. M., Siperstein, G. N., & Bocian, K. M. (1996). The labyrinth of IDEA: School decisions on referred students with subaverage general intelligence. *American Journal of Mental Retardation, 101*, 161–174.

March, J. S., & Leonard, H. L. (1996). Obsessive–compulsive disorder in children and adolescents: A review of the past 10 years. *Journal of the American Academy of Child and Adolescent Psychiatry, 35*, 1265–1273.

Marks, I. M. (1969). *Fears and phobias.* Oxford, UK: Academic Press.

Marks, I. (1988). Blood–injury phobia: A review. *American Journal of Psychiatry, 145*, 1207–1213.

Mash, E. J., & Barkley, R. A. (Eds.). (2009). *Assessment of childhood disorders* (4th ed.). New York: Guilford Press.

Mash, E. J., & Barkley, R. A. (Eds.). (2014). *Child psychopathology* (3rd ed.). New York: Guilford Press.

Max, J. E., & Dunisch, D. L. (1997). Traumatic brain injury in a child psychiatry outpatient clinic: A controlled study. *Journal of the American Academy of Child and Adolescent Psychiatry, 36*, 404–411.

Max, J. E., Robin, D. A., Lindgren, S. D., Smith, W. L., Sato, Y., Mattheis, P. J., et al. (1997). Traumatic brain injury in children and adolescents: Psychiatric disorders at two years. *Journal of the American Academy of Child and Adolescent Psychiatry, 36*, 1278–1285.

Max, J. E., Sharma, A., & Qurashi, M. I. (1997). Traumatic brain injury in a child psychiatric inpatient population: A controlled study. *Journal of the American Academy of Child and Adolescent Psychiatry, 36*, 1595–1601.

Max, J. E., Smith, W. L., Sato, Y., Mattheis, P. J., Castillo, C. S., Lindgren, S. D., et al. (1997). Traumatic brain injury in children and adolescents: Psychiatric disorders in the first three months. *Journal of the American Academy of Child and Adolescent Psychiatry, 36*, 94–102.

McBride, G. M., Willis, J. O., & Dumont, R. (2014). Best practices in applying legal standards for students with disabilities. In P. L. Harrison & A. Thomas (Eds.), *Best practices in school psychology: Foundations* (pp. 421–436). Bethesda, MD: National Association of School Psychologists.

McBurnett, K., Lahey, B. B., & Pfiffner, L. J. (1993). Diagnosis of attention-deficit disorders in DSM-IV: Scientific basis and implications for education. *Exceptional Children, 60*, 108–117.

McGarvey, E. L., Canterbury, R. J., & Waite, D. (1996). Delinquency and family problems in incarcerated adolescents with and without a history of inhalant use. *Addictive Behavior, 21*, 537–542.

McGinnis, E. (1986). *The relationship between psychiatric hospitalization and special education placement.* Unpublished doctoral dissertation, University of Iowa.

McGlashan, T. H. (1988). Adolescent versus adult onset of mania. *American Journal of Psychiatry, 145*, 221–223.

McLaughlin, K. A., Koenen, K. C., Hill, E. D., Petukhova, M., Sampson, N. A., Zaslavsky, A. M., et al. (2013). Trauma exposure and posttraumatic stress disorder in a national sample of adolescents. *Journal of the American Academy of Child and Adolescent Psychiatry, 52,* 815–830.

McNally, R. J. (1993). Stressors that produce posttraumatic stress disorder in children. In J. R. T. Davidson & E. B. Foa (Eds.), *Posttraumatic stress disorder: DSM-IV and beyond* (pp. 57–74). Washington, DC: American Psychiatric Press.

Menolascino, F. J. (1988). Mental illness in the mentally retarded: Diagnostic and treatment issues. In J. A. Stark, F. J. Menolascino, M. H. Albarelli, & V. C. Gray (Eds.), *Mental retardation and mental health: Classification, diagnosis, treatment, services* (pp. 109–123). New York: Springer-Verlag.

Meyer, R. G., & Weaver, C. M. (2006). *The clinician's handbook: Integrated diagnostics, assessment, and intervention in adult and adolescent psychopathology* (5th ed.). Needham Heights, MA: Allyn & Bacon.

Meyers, J. L., & Dick, D. M. (2010). Genetic and environmental risk factors for adolescent-onset substance use disorders. *Child and Adolescent Psychiatric Clinics of North America, 19,* 465–477.

Miller, L. C., Barrett, C. L., & Hampe, E. (1974). Phobias of childhood in a prescientific era. In A. Davids (Ed.), *Child personality and psychopathology: Current topics* (Vol. 1, pp. 89–134). New York: Wiley.

Milne, J. M., Garrison, C. Z., Addy, C. L., McKeown, R. E., Jackson, K. L., Cuffe, S. P., et al. (1995). Frequency of phobic disorder in a community sample of young adolescents. *Journal of the American Academy of Child and Adolescent Psychiatry, 34,* 1202–1211.

Mischel, W. (1968). *Personality and assessment.* New York: Wiley.

Morgan, S. B. (1990). Early childhood autism: Current perspectives on definition, assessment, and treatment. In S. B. Morgan & T. M. Okwumabua (Eds.), *Child and adolescent disorders: Developmental and health psychology perspectives* (pp. 3–45). Hillsdale, NJ: Erlbaum.

Motta, R. W. (1995). Childhood posttraumatic stress disorder and the schools. *Canadian Journal of School Psychology, 11,* 65–78.

Mrazek, D. A. (1994). Psychiatric aspects of somatic disease and disorders. In M. Rutter, E. Taylor, & L. Hersov (Eds.), *Child and adolescent psychiatry: Modern approaches* (pp. 697–710). Oxford, UK: Blackwell.

Namasivayam, A. K., Pukonen, M., Goshulak, D., Yu, V. Y., Kadis, D. S., Kroll, R., et al. (2013). Relationship between speech motor control and speech intelligibility in children with speech sound disorders. *Journal of Communication Disorders, 46,* 264–280.

National Institute on Alcohol Abuse and Alcoholism. (2011). *Alcohol screening and brief intervention for youth: A practitioner's guide.* Rockville, MD: National Institute on Alcohol Abuse and Alcoholism Publications. Retrieved from *http://pubs.niaaa.nih.gov/publications/Practitioner/YouthGuide/YouthGuideOrderForm.htm.*

Newcorn, J. H., & Strain, J. (1992). Adjustment disorder in children and adolescents. *Journal of the American Academy of Child and Adolescent Psychiatry, 31,* 318–327.

Nordyke, N. S., Baer, D. M., Etzel, B. C., & LeBlanc, J. M. (1977). Implications of the stereotyping of modification of sex role. *Journal of Applied Behavior Analysis, 10*, 553–557.

Novins, D. K., Bechtold, D. W., Sack, W. H., Thompson, J., Carter, D. R., & Manson, S. M. (1997). The DSM-IV outline for cultural formulation: A critical demonstration with American Indian children. *Journal of the American Academy of Child and Adolescent Psychiatry, 36*, 1244–1251.

Nurcombe, B., Mitchell, W., Begtrup, R., Tramontana, M., LaBarbera, J., & Pruitt, J. (1996). Dissociative hallucinosis and allied conditions. In F. R. Volkmar (Ed.), *Psychoses and pervasive developmental disorders in childhood and adolescence* (pp. 107–128). Washington, DC: American Psychiatric Press.

Oakland, T. (1992). School dropouts: Characteristics and prevention. *Applied and Preventive Psychology, 1*, 201–208.

Palla, B., & Litt, I. R. (1988). Medical complications of eating disorders in adolescents. *Pediatrics, 81*, 613–623.

Pauls, D. L., Alsobrook, J. P., II, Goodman, W., Rasmussen, S., & Leckman, J. F. (1995). A family study of obsessive–compulsive disorder. *American Journal of Psychiatry, 152*, 76–84.

Pavkov, T. W., Lewis, D. A., & Lyons, J. S. (1989). Psychiatric diagnosis and racial bias: An empirical investigation. *Professional Psychology: Research and Practice, 20*, 364–368.

Pfeffer, C. R. (1992). Relationship between depression and suicidal behavior. In M. Shafii & S. L. Shafii (Eds.), *Clinical guide to depression in children and adolescents* (pp. 115–126). Washington, DC: American Psychiatric Press.

Pfefferbaum, B. (1997). Posttraumatic stress disorder in children: A review of the past 10 years. *Journal of the American Academy of Child and Adolescent Psychiatry, 36*, 1503–1511.

Pietrini, P., Dani, A., Furey, M. L., Alexander, G. E., Freo, U., Grady, C. L., et al. (1997). Low glucose metabolism during brain stimulation in older Down's syndrome subjects at risk for Alzheimer's disease prior to dementia. *American Journal of Psychiatry, 154*, 1063–1069.

Pilowsky, D. (1986). Problems in determining the presence of hallucinations in children. In D. Pilowsky & W. Chambers (Eds.), *Hallucinations in children* (pp. 1–16). Washington, DC: American Psychiatric Press.

Pliszka, S. R. (2015). Comorbid psychiatric disorders in children with ADHD. In R. A. Barkley (Ed.), *Attention-deficit/hyperactivity disorder: A handbook for diagnosis and treatment* (4th ed., pp. 140–168). New York: Guilford Press.

Power, T. J., & DuPaul, G. J. (1996a). Attention-deficit/hyperactivity disorder: The reemergence of subtypes. *School Psychology Review, 25*, 284–296.

Power, T. J., & DuPaul, G. J. (1996b). Implications of DSM-IV for the practice of school psychology: Introduction to the mini-series. *School Psychology Review, 25*, 255–258.

Putnam, F. W. (1996). Posttraumatic stress disorder in children and adolescents.

In L. J. Dickstein, M. B. Riba, & J. M. Oldham (Eds.), *Review of psychiatry* (Vol. 15, pp. 447–468). Washington, DC: American Psychiatric Press.

Putnam, F. W., Helmers, K., & Trickett, P. K. (1993). Development, reliability and validity of a child dissociation scale. *Child Abuse and Neglect, 17,* 731–741.

Putnam, C. T., & Kirkpatrick, J. T. (2005, May). Juvenile firesetting: A research overview. *Juvenile Justice Bulletin.* Retrieved November 30, 2014, from *www.ojp.usdoj.gov.*

Rapee, R. M., Schniering, C. A., & Hudson, J. L. (2009). Anxiety disorders during childhood and adolescence: Origins and treatment. *Annual Review of Clinical Psychology, 5,* 311–341.

Rapoport, J. L. (1997). What is known about childhood schizophrenia? *Harvard Mental Health Letter, 14,* 8.

Reeves, R. R., & Bullen, J. A. (1995). Mnemonics for ten DSM-IV disorders. *Journal of Nervous and Mental Disease, 183,* 550–551.

Reid, R. (1995). Assessment of ADHD with culturally different groups: The use of behavioral rating scales. *School Psychology Review, 24,* 537–560.

Reiss, S. (1994). Issues in defining mental retardation. *American Journal on Mental Retardation, 99,* 1–7.

Rekers, G. A., & Lovaas, I. O. (1974). Behavioral treatment of deviant sex role behaviors in a male child. *Journal of Applied Behavior Analysis, 7,* 173–190.

Rind, B., Tromovitch, P., & Bauserman, R. (1998). A meta-analytic examination of assumed properties of child sexual abuse using college samples. *Psychological Bulletin, 124,* 22–53.

Rivara, J. B., Jaffe, K. M., Fay, G. C., Polissar, N. L., Martin, K. M., Shurtleff, H. A., et al. (1993). Family functioning and injury severity as predictors of child functioning one year following traumatic brain injury. *Archives of Physical Medicine and Rehabilitation, 74,* 1047–1055.

Roberts, M. A. (1990). A behavioral observation method for differentiating hyperactive and aggressive boys. *Journal of Abnormal Child Psychology, 18,* 131–142.

Robins, L. R. (1991). Conduct disorder. *Journal of Child Psychiatry and Psychology, 32,* 193–212.

Rourke, B. P. (1989). *Nonverbal learning disabilities: The syndrome and the model.* New York: Guilford Press.

Russell, A. T., Bott, L., & Sammons, C. (1989). The phenomenology of schizophrenia occurring in childhood. *Journal of the American Academy of Child and Adolescent Psychiatry, 28,* 399–407.

Rutter, M. (1981). Psychological sequelae of brain damage in children. *American Journal of Psychiatry, 138,* 1533–1544.

Ryan, N. D., Puig-Antich, J., Ambrosini, P., Rabinovich, H., Robinson, D., Nelson, B., et al. (1987). The clinical picture of major depression in children and adolescents. *Archives of General Psychiatry, 44,* 854–861.

Sabatino, D. A., & Vance, H. B. (1994). Is the diagnosis of attention-deficit/

hyperactivity disorder meaningful? *Psychology in the Schools, 31*, 188–196.

Sands, R., Tricker, J., Sherman, C., Armatas, C., & Maschette, W. (1997). Disordered eating patterns, body image, self-esteem, and physical activity in preadolescent school children. *International Journal of Eating Disorders, 21*, 159–166.

Schalock, R. L., Borthwick-Duffy, S. A., Bradley, V. J., Buntinx, W. H. E., Coulter, D. L., Craig, E. M., et al. (2010). *Intellectual disability: Definition, classification, and systems of supports* (11th ed.). Washington, DC: American Association on Intellectual and Developmental Disabilities.

Scheeringa, M. S., Zeanah, C. H., & Cohen, J. A. (2011). PTSD in children and adolescents: Toward an empirically based algorithm. *Depression and Anxiety, 28*, 770–782.

Schmidt, C. W., Jr., Yowell, R. K., & Jaffe, E. (2010). *Procedure coding handbook for psychiatrists.* Washington, DC: American Psychiatric Publishing.

Schulte, I. E., & Petermann, F. (2011). Somatoform disorders: 30 years of debate about criteria! What about children and adolescents? *Journal of Psychosomatic Research, 70*, 218–228.

Schwarz, E. D., & Kowalski, J. M. (1991). Posttraumatic stress disorder after a school shooting: Effects of symptom threshold selection and diagnosis by DSM-III, DSM-III-R, or proposed DSM-IV. *American Journal of Psychiatry, 148*, 592–597.

Scott, S. (1994). Mental retardation. In M. Rutter, E. Taylor, & L. Hersov (Eds.), *Child and adolescent psychiatry: Modern approaches* (3rd ed., pp. 616–646). Oxford, UK: Blackwell.

Scotti, J. R., Morris, T. L., McNeil, C. B., & Hawkins, R. P. (1996). DSM-IV and disorders of childhood and adolescence: Can structural criteria be functional? *Journal of Consulting and Clinical Psychology, 64*, 1177–1191.

Shamsie, J., & Hluchy, C. (1991). Youth with conduct disorder: A challenge to be met. *Canadian Journal of Psychiatry, 36*, 405–414.

Shaywitz, S. E., Escobar, M. E., Shaywitz, B. A., Fletcher, J. M., & Makuch, R. (1990). Evidence that dyslexia may represent the lower tail of a normal distribution of reading ability. *New England Journal of Medicine, 326*, 145–150.

Shaywitz, S. E., Shaywitz, B. A., Fletcher, J. M., & Escobar, M. E. (1990). Prevalence of reading disability in boys and girls: Results of the Connecticut longitudinal study. *Journal of the American Medical Association, 264*, 998–1002.

Siegel, M., & Barthel, R. P. (1986). Conversion disorders on a child psychiatry consultation service. *Psychosomatics, 27*, 201–204.

Silk, J. S., Nath, S. R., Siegel, L. R., & Kendall, P. C. (2000). Conceptualizing mental disorders in children: Where have we been and where are we going? *Development and Psychopathology, 12*, 713–735.

Simeon, J. G. (1989). Depressive disorders in children and adolescents. *Psychiatry Journal of the University of Ottawa, 14*, 356–361.

Skagerberg, E., Parkinson, R., & Carmichael, P. (2013). Self-harming thoughts and behaviors in a group of children and adolescents with gender dysphoria. *International Journal of Transgenderism, 14*, 86–92.

Skirbekk, B., Hansen, B. H., Oerbeck, B., & Kristensen, H. (2011). The relationship between sluggish cognitive tempo, subtypes of attention-deficit/hyperactivity disorder, and anxiety disorders. *Journal of Abnormal Child Psychology, 39*, 513–525.

Skodol, A. E. (1989). *Problems in differential diagnosis: From DSM-III to DSM-III-R in clinical practice*. Washington, DC: American Psychiatric Press.

Slater, E. J., & Bassett, S. S. (1988). Adolescents with closed head injuries: A report of initial cognitive deficits. *American Journal of Diseases of Children, 142*, 1048–1051.

Small, R. F. (1991). *Maximizing third-party reimbursement in your mental health practice*. Sarasota, FL: Professional Resource Exchange.

Smart, D., Sanson, A., & Prior, M. (1996). Connections between reading disability and behavior problems: Testing temporal and causal hypotheses. *Journal of Abnormal Child Psychology, 24*, 363–383.

Spack, N. P., Edwards-Leeper, L., Feldman, H. A., Leibowitz, S., Mandel, F., Diamond, D. A., et al. (2012). Children and adolescents with gender identity disorder referred to a pediatric medical center. *Pediatrics, 129*, 418–425.

State, M. W., King, B. H., & Dykens, E. (1997). Mental retardation: A review of the past 10 years: Part II. *Journal of the American Academy of Child and Adolescent Psychiatry, 36*, 1664–1671.

Stein, D. J. (1993). Cross-cultural psychiatry and the DSM-IV. *Comprehensive Psychiatry, 34*, 322–329.

Steiner, H., & Lock, J. (1998). Anorexia nervosa and bulimia in children and adolescents: A review of the past 10 years. *Journal of the American Academy of Child and Adolescent Psychiatry, 37*, 352–359.

Steinhausen, H. C., & Juzi, C. (1996). Elective mutism: An analysis of 100 cases. *Journal of the American Academy of Child and Adolescent Psychiatry, 35*, 606–614.

Strauss, C. C., Lease, C. A., Last, C. G., & Francis, G. (1988). Overanxious disorder: An examination of developmental differences. *Journal of Abnormal Child Psychology, 16*, 433–443.

Strub, R. L., & Black, F. W. (1988). *Neurobehavioral disorders: A clinical approach*. Philadelphia: Davis.

Substance Abuse and Mental Health Services Administration. (2015). National Registry of Evidence-based Programs and Practices (NREPP). Retrieved March 22, 2015, from *www.nrepp.samhsa.gov*.

Suveg, C., Aschenbrand, S. G., & Kendall, P. C. (2005). Separation anxiety disorder, panic disorder, and school refusal. *Child and Adolescent Psychiatric Clinics of North America, 14*, 773–795.

Swedo, S. E., Leonard, H. L., Mittleman, B. B., Allen, A. J., Rapoport, J. L.,

Dow, S. P., et al. (1997). Identification of children with pediatric autoimmune neuropsychiatric disorders associated with streptococcal infections by a marker associated with rheumatic fever. *American Journal of Psychiatry, 154*, 110–112.

Swedo, S. E., Rapoport, J. L., Leonard, H., Lenane, M., & Cheslow, D. (1989). Obsessive–compulsive disorder in children and adolescents: Clinical phenomenology of 70 consecutive cases. *Archives of General Psychiatry, 46*, 335–341.

Swendsen, J., Burstein, M., Case, B., Conway, K. P., Dierker, L., He, J., et al. (2012). Use and abuse of alcohol and illicit drugs in U.S. adolescents. *Archives of General Psychiatry, 69*, 390–398.

Szymanski, L. S. (1994). Mental retardation and mental health: Concepts, aetiology and incidence. In N. Bouras (Ed.), *Mental health in mental retardation: Recent advances and practices* (pp. 19–33). Cambridge, UK: Cambridge University Press.

Thornton, C., & Russell, J. (1997). Obsessive–compulsive comorbidity in the dieting disorders. *International Journal of Eating Disorders, 21*, 83–87.

Thorpy, M. J. (2012). Classification of sleep disorders. *Neurotherapeutics, 9*, 687–701.

Tobin, R. M., Schneider, W. J., & Landau, S. (2014). Best practices in the assessment of youth with attention-deficit/hyperactivity disorder within a multitiered services framework. In P. L. Harrison & A. Thomas (Eds.), *Best practices in school psychology: Data-based and collaborative decision making* (pp. 391–404). Bethesda, MD: National Association of School Psychologists.

Tsai, L. Y. (2014). Impact of DSM-5 on epidemiology of autism spectrum disorder. *Research in Autism Spectrum Disorders, 8*, 1454–1470.

Tumuluru, R., Yaylayan, S., Weller, E. B., & Weller, R. A. (1996). Affective psychoses: I. Major depression with psychosis. In F. R. Volkmar (Ed.), *Psychoses and pervasive developmental disorders in childhood and adolescence* (pp. 49–69). Washington, DC: American Psychiatric Press.

Turkat, I. D. (1990). *The personality disorders: A psychological approach to clinical management*. New York: Pergamon Press.

U.S. Department of Education. (2015). Individuals with Disabilities Education Improvement Act of 2004. Retrieved March 16, 2015, from *www.gpo.gov/fdsys/pkg/PLAW-108publ446/html/PLAW-108publ446.htm.*

Üstün, T. B., Chatterji, S., Kostanjsek, N., Rehm, J., Kennedy, C., Epping-Jordan, J., et al. (2010). Developing the World Health Organization Disability Assessment Schedule 2.0. *Bulletin of the World Health Organization, 88*, 815–823.

Vitiello, B., & Stoff, D. M. (1997). Subtypes of aggression and their relevance to child psychiatry. *Journal of the American Academy of Child and Adolescent Psychiatry, 36*, 307–315.

Wakefield, J. C. (2013). DSM-5: An overview of changes and controversies. *Clinical Social Work Journal, 41*, 139–154.

Walter, A. L., & Carter, A. S. (1997). Gilles de la Tourette's syndrome in childhood: A guide for school professionals. *School Psychology Review, 26*, 28–46.

Weinberg, W. A., & Brumback, R. A. (1976). Mania in childhood: Case studies and literature review. *American Journal of Diseases of Children, 130*, 380–385.

Werry, J. S. (1996). Childhood schizophrenia. In F. R. Volkmar (Ed.), *Psychoses and pervasive developmental disorders in childhood and adolescence* (pp. 1–56). Washington, DC: American Psychiatric Press.

Westen, D., Ludolph, P., Lerner, H., Ruffins, S., & Wiss, F. C. (1990). Object relations in borderline adolescents. *Journal of the American Academy of Child and Adolescent Psychiatry, 29*, 338–348.

Whitaker, S., & Read, S. (2006). The prevalence of psychiatric disorders among people with intellectual disabilities: An analysis of the literature. *Journal of Applied Research in Intellectual Disabilities, 19*(4), 330–345.

Wiederman, M. W., & Pryor, T. (1996). Substance use and impulsive behaviors among adolescents with eating disorders. *Addictive Behaviors, 21*, 269–272.

Wolfe, B. E. (1979). Behavioral treatment of childhood gender disorders. *Behavior Modification, 4*, 550–575.

Wolpe, J. (1990). *The practice of behavior therapy* (4th ed.). New York: Pergamon Press.

Woolgar, M., & Scott, S. (2014). The negative consequences of over-diagnosing attachment disorders in adopted children: The importance of comprehensive formulations. *Clinical Child Psychology and Psychiatry, 19*, 355–366.

World Health Organization. (1977). *Manual of the International Statistical Classification of Diseases, Injuries, and Causes of Death* (9th rev., 2 vols.). Geneva, Switzerland: Author.

World Health Organization. (1992). *Manual of the International Statistical Classification of Diseases and Related Health Problems* (10th rev., 3 vols.). Geneva, Switzerland: Author.

World Health Organization. (1993). *The ICD-10 classification of mental and behavioural disorders: Diagnostic criteria for research.* Geneva, Switzerland: Author.

Wulfert, E., Greenway, D. E., & Dougher, M. J. (1996). A logical functional analysis of reinforcement-based disorders: Alcoholism and pedophilia. *Journal of Consulting and Clinical Psychology, 64*, 1140–1151.

Wynick, S., Hobson, R. P., & Jones, R. B. (1997). Psychogenic disorders of vision in childhood ("visual conversion reactions"): Perspectives from adolescence: A research note. *Journal of Child Psychiatry and Psychology, 38*, 375–379.

Yaylayan, S., Tumuluru, R., Weller, E. B., & Weller, R. A. (1996). Affective psychoses: II. Bipolar disorder with psychosis. In F. R. Volkmar (Ed.), *Psychoses and pervasive developmental disorders in childhood and adolescence* (pp. 71–88). Washington, DC: American Psychiatric Press.

Yoo, J. H., Valdovinos, M. G., & Schroeder, S. R. (2012). The epidemiology of psychopathology in people with intellectual disability: A forty-year review. In R. M. Hodapp (Ed.), *International review of research in developmental disabilities* (Vol. 42, pp. 31–56). San Diego, CA: Elsevier Science.

Yorbik, O., Birmaher, B., Axelson, D., Williamson, D. E., & Ryan, N. D. (2004). Clinical characteristics of depressive symptoms in children and adolescents with major depressive disorder. *Journal of Clinical Psychiatry, 65,* 1654–1659.

Yorkston, K. M., Jaffe, K. M., Polissar, N. L., Liao, S., & Fay, G. C. (1997). Written language production and neuropsychological function in children with traumatic brain injury. *Archives of Physical Medicine and Rehabilitation, 78,* 1096–1102.

Young, J. E. (1990). *Cognitive therapy for personality disorders: A schema-focused approach.* Sarasota, FL: Professional Resources Exchange.

Zoccolillo, M., Meyers, J., & Assiter, S. (1997). Conduct disorder, substance dependence, and adolescent motherhood. *American Journal of Orthopsychiatry, 67,* 152–157.

Zucker, K. J. (1990). Treatment of gender identity disorders in children. In R. Blanchard & B. W. Steiner (Eds.), *Clinical management of gender identity disorders in children and adults* (pp. 25–47). Washington, DC: American Psychiatric Association.

Zumeta, R. O., Zirkel, P. A., & Danielson, L. (2014). Identifying specific learning disabilities: Legislation, regulation, and court decisions. *Topics in Language Disorders, 34,* 8–24.

Index

Page numbers in italic denote a figure or table.

N

P